EXERCISE BALL
for BEGINNERS

CHRISSIE GALLAGHER-MUNDY

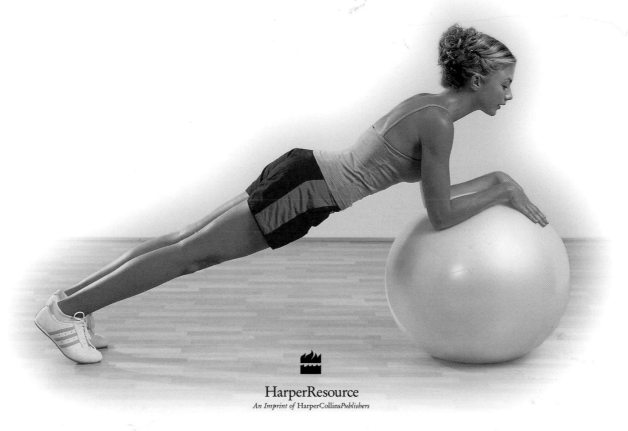

HarperResource
An Imprint of HarperCollinsPublishers

CREATED AND PRODUCED BY:
Carroll & Brown Limited
20 Lonsdale Road
London NW6 6RD

FIRST PUBLISHED IN THE USA IN 2004 BY:
HarperResource, an imprint of HarperCollins Publishers

Project Editor: Kirsten Chapman
Art Editor: Justin Ford
Production: Karol Davies, Nigel Reed, Nicky Rein, Paul Stradling
Photographer: Jules Selmes
Photographic Assistant: David Yems

For information address HarperCollins Publishers, Inc.
10 East 53rd Street, New York, NY 10022.

HarperCollins books may be purchased for educational, business, or sales promotional use. For information, please write: Special Markets Department, HarperCollins Publishers, Inc. 10 East 53rd Street, New York, NY 10022.

FIRST U.S. EDITION

ISBN 0–06–058595–1

The exercises in this book are safe if performed as described, but you should consult your doctor before beginning this or any other exercise program, especially if you have an existing medical condition. Neither the exercises nor the information given with them are intended to replace medical advice. If you have any concerns about your health, consult your doctor. Neither the author nor the publishers shall be liable or responsible for any loss, injury, or damage allegedly arising from any information or suggestion in this book.

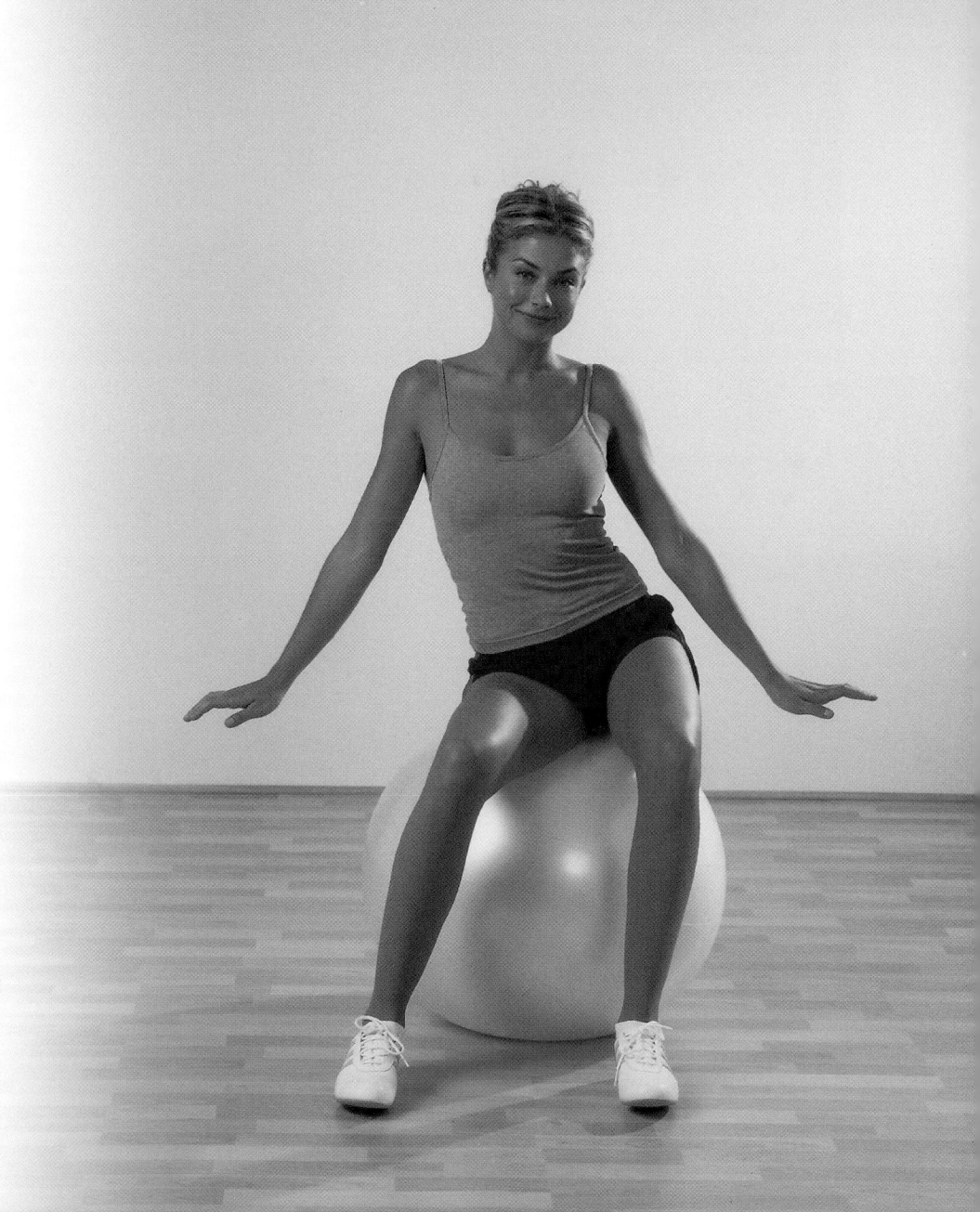

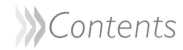

Contents

⟫Introduction: Why the Ball?

A piece of equipment that is fun as well as effective is worth a lot. The exercise ball was originally developed in the 1960s as a toy for children, but soon physiotherapists in Switzerland discovered that it could be a useful tool to help patients recover from injuries—which explains why you might sometimes hear it called a "Swiss ball." Through seminars and clinical workshops, the exercise ball's popularity spread, until coaches and personal trainers started using it to condition elite athletes, and before long, the general public. Now the exercise ball is one of the most popular and respected pieces of gym equipment among fitness professionals and enthusiasts alike—and not without good reason.

How does the ball work?

The exercise ball's effectiveness is largely due to the fact that it provides an unstable base on which to exercise. Balance is neglected in many exercise programs, yet any moves that require balance recruit many more muscles than those in which you're standing squarely on two feet. When you sit, lie, or rest your legs on the ball you need to engage the muscles of your core—your stomach, sides, back, and buttocks—in order to keep your body and the ball in place. This means that not only do you tone these areas, but also you strengthen the muscles that support the spine. In the long term this can help improve your posture and prevent back problems.

The ball also provides a very versatile tool for toning and strengthening individual muscle groups. As with a weight bench, you can lie on top of the ball to isolate and work specific muscles, including those in your arms, legs, shoulders, and back. Yet the ball is much more comfortable than a bench, since it molds to the shape of your body. The large, curved surface of the ball also allows you to position your body on different planes, so you can tip yourself up or down to increase or decrease the intensity of an exercise. And, because you can wrap your body around the ball, you can get a far greater range of movement than you can on the floor, thus improving the quality of your exercises, particularly those for your abdominals or back.

Another benefit of the ball is that it moves. If lifting weights or using resistance bands aren't your thing, you can use the traction of rolling the ball along the floor to help tone your muscles. Because you can

HOW TO USE THIS BOOK

This book has a folding base so you can stand it up next to you while you work through the program. Read the Introduction (pages 4–19) thoroughly before beginning any of the exercises; this tells you how to exercise safely and how to get the most out of your workouts. Then follow the exercises by flipping the pages: the top page gives you background information about the exercise and the bottom page shows you how to do it.

For an all-over workout, do all the exercises in the Core Training, Toning, and Stretching sections, as well as a warm-up and cool-down. This should last about an hour and a half. If you don't have that long, turn to Timed Routines (see page 88) for a shorter workout. Read the annotations on the top page pictures to be sure you get the most out of the exercise, and always check the Safety First boxes, particularly if you have any injuries.

roll the ball in any direction, it's easy to make minute adjustments to your form. If you stretch too far, you can simply roll back to a more comfortable position. Or if you are doing an exercise that might put

ADDITIONAL BENEFITS OF THE BALL

- *Working your core muscles regularly will remind you to maintain good posture in everyday life.*
- *Exercising or simply sitting on the ball stimulates tiny balance receptors in your tendons and muscles. Using these regularly improves your stability and coordination, helping prevent trips and falls.*
- *Doing a nonstop routine on the ball will raise your heart rate, so working out regularly can improve your heart health and circulation.*
- *Stretching and improving your flexibility will keep you more fit as you get older.*
- *Toning your muscles will help with weight loss, as your muscles continue to burn calories even after you've finished your workout. Good posture will make you look instantly slimmer.*
- *Rolling around on the ball is incredibly relaxing—as well as a fun way to release tension and help you wind down at the end of a long day.*

pressure on your joints, like a lunge or squat, you can use the support of the ball to help you move slowly and safely, without fear of strain or injury.

Who does the ball suit?

Because the ball is so flexible, sensitive, and safe, it's great for people of all abilities and levels of fitness. If you're new to exercise, you'll find that it's fun and easy to use. Once you've bought your ball and found a space to exercise—which can be in the comfort of your own home or backyard— you're ready to go. And, if you stick to your exercise program, you'll quickly see the results: a stronger, more toned body and better flexibility, posture, and balance. If you already play sports or follow a

workout program, an exercise ball is the perfect complement to almost any routine. If you regularly cycle, swim, walk, or do any form of cardiovascular exercise, then the ball provides an interesting way to work on the other key fitness areas of strength and flexibility. If you currently practice yoga or pilates, you can use the ball to help you stretch farther, as well as to focus on building muscle tone and strength. If you do any sports that involve using your back and torso muscles, such as golf or tennis, you'll soon find that improving your core strength (see page 21) can be a great boost to your game. Whatever you're looking to achieve, the ball will certainly bring a new dimension to your workout.

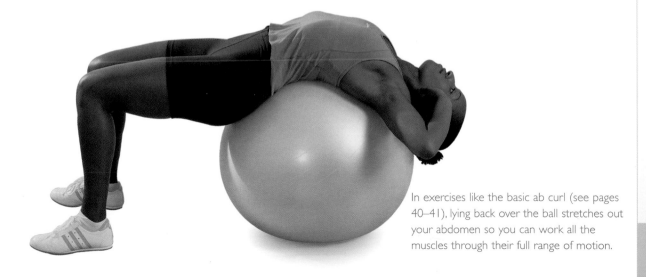

In exercises like the basic ab curl (see pages 40–41), lying back over the ball stretches out your abdomen so you can work all the muscles through their full range of motion.

⟫ A Good Program

Sports and health professionals agree that there are three main elements of fitness: strength, flexibility, and cardiovascular health. Many people who exercise regularly tend to concentrate on only one or two of these elements, perhaps because they have a specific goal—such as building muscle or losing weight—or because they prefer a particular sport or activity. But if you want to improve your overall health and quality of life, along with looking and feeling good, then you need to design a program that includes all three.

Toning and strengthening

When fitness experts talk about "strength" they are referring to power and endurance in your muscles. For example, you need muscular power to perform a short but strenuous action, like lifting a heavy suitcase off a baggage belt, whereas you need muscular endurance to sustain an activity, such as carrying the groceries from the store to your car. Building strength not only helps you perform everyday activities with ease and reduces your risk of injury, but also helps you shape up and look great— a strong muscle is also a toned muscle.

An exercise ball is a versatile tool for strength work, and in the Core Training and Toning sections you'll find exercises for all the major muscle groups. For the best results, include all or at least a variety of these exercises in each of your workouts. Even if you want to focus on just one

(cont.)

With many toning exercises, such as the back toner (see pages 38–39), you can vary your position to make it easier or harder—note your progression over the weeks.

HOW OFTEN SHOULD YOU EXERCISE?

The more regularly you exercise, the sooner you'll see results and the better they'll be. Aim for three workouts per week, and you should start to notice a difference in your physique within six weeks. Try not to do the same core training or toning exercises on subsequent days—your muscles need a chance to rest. If on a particular day you don't have time to do all

the exercises, the timed routines section will help you plan a good workout (see pages 88–95). Don't forget to include two or three sessions of cardiovascular exercise in your weekly routine; if you do one before your workout, it can serve as your warm-up.

area, you'll get better results from toning your whole body. This is because building muscles increases your overall metabolic rate—the rate at which you burn calories, even when you're just sitting in a chair. Keep in mind also that although doing hundreds of abdominal crunches will help firm up your stomach muscles, it won't get rid of the layer of fat that covers them. To lose fat, you need to combine your strength exercises with cardiovascular exercise and a healthy diet (see pages 8–9).

Stretching

Being flexible means having the full range of movement in your joints and muscles. The more flexible you are, the better you can reach a book off a high shelf, bend down and tie your shoelaces, or turn to look over

As a stretching tool, the ball is highly versatile, allowing you to stretch the parts you wouldn't normally reach.

your shoulder. As we get older and become less active, our muscles and tendons tighten and we lose some of our mobility. The same thing can happen, too, if you exercise regularly but don't stretch. After lifting weights, for example, your muscle fibers tend to contract and shorten, so decreasing your flexibility.

Stretching regularly, and particularly after exercise, counteracts these effects and lengthens the muscles. In the short term, this releases tension, helps prevent aches and injuries, and is very relaxing.

In the long term, stretching gives you a longer, leaner look, improves your mobility and posture, and helps you stay active later in life.

Stretching on the ball is easy. For all-around fitness, include exercises from the stretching section in each of your ball workouts, or, if you regularly do strength training or cardiovascular exercise, stretch on the ball to cool down after your workouts. Just make sure you read all the technique and safety tips before you start, and keep in mind that a safe stretch is a gentle stretch. If it hurts, stop.

SAFETY FIRST

Warm up with 5–10 minutes of gentle cardiovascular activity at the beginning of every workout—even if just doing toning or stretching exercises—to prevent injury to your joints, muscles, and tendons. Finish each workout with a cool-down consisting of gentle stretches and relaxation exercises (see pages 14–19).

≫A Good Program (2)

Cardiovascular exercise

Also called aerobic training, this refers to exercises in which your muscles use oxygen as a fuel. To increase the supply of oxygen-rich blood to your muscles, your heart pumps faster and more forcefully. Cardio-vascular exercise is carried out over a sustained period and includes activities like jogging, cycling, and swimming. It doesn't include short bursts of activity, such as sprinting, in which your body can't keep up with your muscles' demand for oxygen and you quickly become exhausted.

Regular cardiovascular exercise is vital to a good fitness program. Pushing your heart slightly harder each time you work out makes it stronger and more efficient. Over time, this means that not only can your body cope with higher levels of exertion, but also that your resting heart rate decreases, putting less strain on your cardiovascular system (heart, lungs, and blood vessels). This, in turn, lowers your blood pressure and reduces your risk of heart disease.

Cardiovascular exercise has many other benefits besides heart health. It is the key to reducing fat, because your body draws on its reserves of sugar and fat for energy. It helps you breathe better, as it strengthens the muscles around your lungs, and the lungs become more efficient at transferring oxygen to your blood. It also helps you sleep, improves concentration, helps you cope better with stress, and releases serotonin—a naturally occurring chemical that makes you feel happy. For all these reasons and more, build cardiovascular exercise into your routine.

If you do a sequence of exercises on the ball without stopping, you will raise your heart rate and burn calories. Supplement your ball workouts with regular cardiovascular exercise, however. Any activity that raises your heart rate and brings you out in a light sweat—including walking, dancing, or aerobics classes—will be good for you, as long as you do it regularly: at least three times a week, for at least 30 minutes each time.

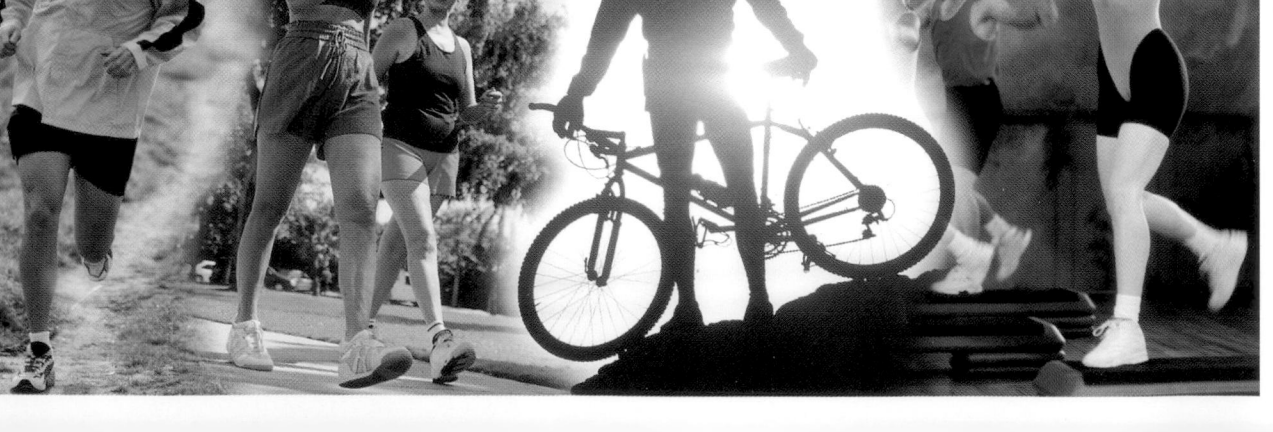

When you do cardiovascular activities, you'll perspire and your heart will beat faster, but you should feel comfortable. If you're working so hard you can't talk, slow down.

Healthy diet and nutrition

A good program doesn't stop at exercise. For optimum health, you need to eat a diet that's balanced, which means eating the right proportions of the right foods.

- Just over a third of your daily intake should come from breads, cereals, pasta, and potatoes. These provide energy and fiber, which keeps your digestive system in good working order. Where possible, choose unrefined versions, such as brown rice or pasta or wholewheat bread, as these contain plenty of fiber and give you a slow, sustained energy release.
- Fruits and vegetables should make up another third of your intake, and this means at least five servings a day. Fruits and vegetables contain fiber as well as essential vitamins and minerals, which keep your body systems functioning properly, maintain healthy bones and teeth, and transport nutrients around your body. Aim to eat lots of fresh fruits and vegetables of different types and colors.
- Protein foods—such as meat, poultry, fish, beans, nuts, and seeds—should make up a smaller proportion of your daily intake: about two to three servings a day. Aim to eat oily fish such as salmon or mackerel twice a week.

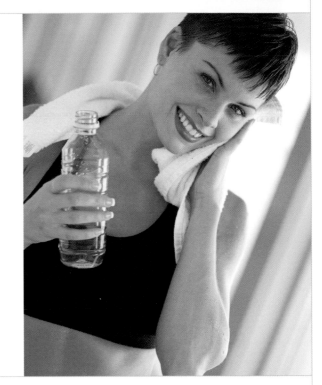

WHY DRINK WATER?

- *When you exercise, your body temperature rises and you sweat. Regular sips of water help keep you cool and replace lost fluids.*
- *Water helps transport food through the digestive tract and flushes out waste and toxins.*
- *Water can help you lose weight, as it assists the fat-burning process and decreases your appetite, but contains no calories.*
- *If you don't give your body enough water, it starts to hold onto it and you get fluid retention. Drinking water reverses this.*
- *Healthy skin has a high water content—around 10–20 percent. Drink plenty for a youthful glow.*
- *Headaches and lack of concentration are signs of dehydration. Drink water to relieve them.*

- You only need about two to three servings of milk and dairy foods each day. Choose low-fat versions where possible.
- Fats, oils, and sweet foods should make up the smallest proportion of your diet. Limit your intake of cookies, chocolate, and sugary foods, as well as saturated fats (found in butter, fatty meat, cheese, and pastries). Opt for unsaturated fats, which include olive oil, vegetable oils, nuts and nut oils, and oily fish.

- Finally, keep up your fluid intake. Drink at least eight 8-ounce (250-ml) glasses of fluids a day, including water, fruit juices, and herbal teas. You need more when you're exercising, so take frequent sips of water, before, during, and after a workout. Limit your overall intake of caffeine and alcohol.

≫ Before You Begin

Whatever your current level of fitness, exercising on the ball can be of great benefit to your health. To make sure you are getting the most out of your workouts and that you're not putting yourself at risk of injury, however, always begin a new program of exercise slowly, and take time to choose your ball and learn how to use it correctly.

Health matters

If you haven't exercised in the last three months, consult your doctor to check that he or she approves of you beginning a program of exercise at home. If you already exercise regularly and are fit and well, then you should be able to work through this book with confidence. As with all new pieces of equipment, treat the ball with caution until you get used to working with it.

After the first few workouts, you may experience some stiffness because you are using your muscles in a new way. The way to reduce this is to use the ball regularly—any aches should ease in a few days, and you'll soon find that exercising with the ball increases your flexibility and helps reduce muscle tension. However, if an ache persists or if you experience a sharp or sudden pain during your workout, stop exercising and contact your doctor as soon as possible.

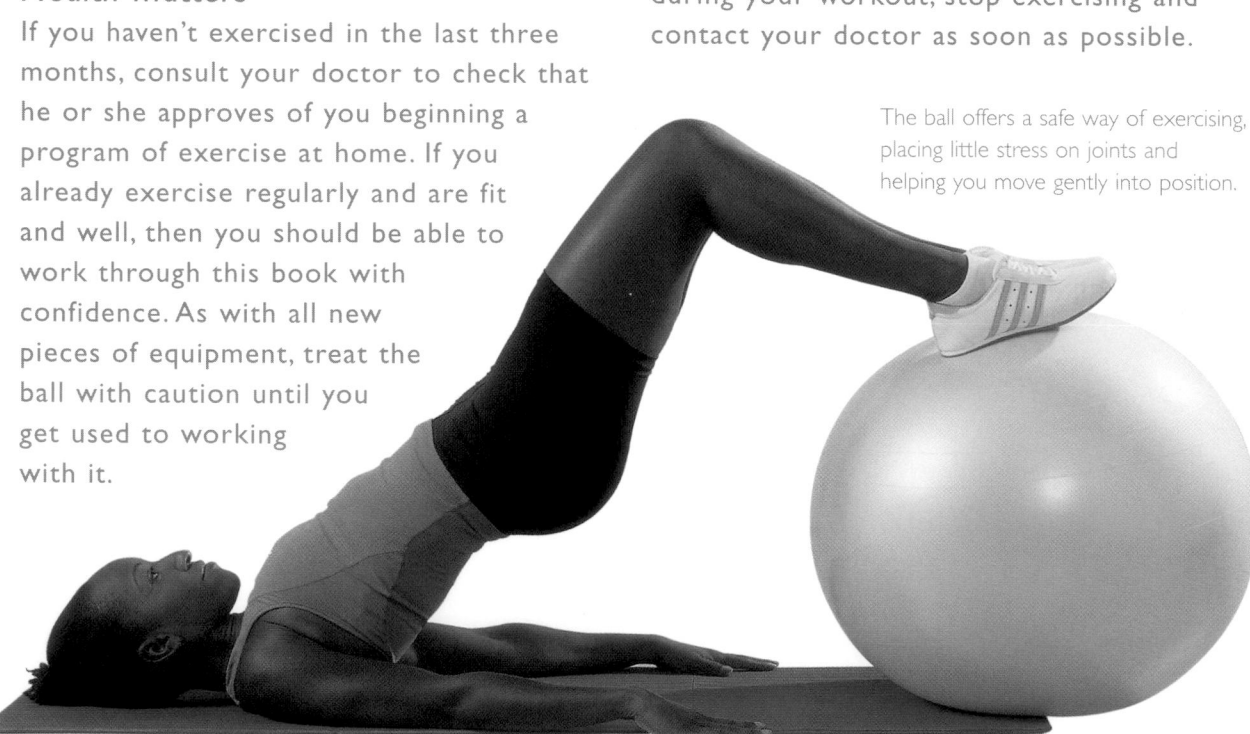

The ball offers a safe way of exercising, placing little stress on joints and helping you move gently into position.

SAFETY FIRST

Consult your doctor before you exercise if you have any of the following:

• cardiovascular disease
• osteoporosis
• episodes of dizziness
• arthritis
• back pain
• or if you are pregnant

During your workout stop exercising and contact your doctor if you experience:

• pain or discomfort
• dizziness, faintness, or nausea
• shortness of breath
• rapid heart rate
• excessive sweating

Choosing a ball that's right for you

With the variety of names—gym ball, Swiss ball, fit ball, stability ball, resistance ball—and a variety of sizes, it may seem that you have too many choices when selecting your exercise ball. You do need to make sure that the ball you buy is right for you, though.

The most important thing is that the ball is the right size for your height so that you can maintain the correct position throughout your exercises; generally speaking, the taller you are, the larger the ball you need—see the chart below to find out the diameter of ball you'll need. When you sit centrally on the inflated ball, you should be able to sit with your feet flat and your hips and knees at a 90-degree angle (see the basic sit position on page 13).

Exercise balls are usually quite inexpensive, but it's worth making sure you get a good quality ball. A textured surface can prevent slipping and a burst-resistant ball is slightly safer. If punctured, some cheap balls may burst suddenly, like a balloon popping; a burst-resistant ball will deflate slowly preventing you from falling flat on the floor. Some balls even have a burst rating; you'll see something like "burst resistant to 285 lb" on the label. The higher the rating, the tougher the ball, but you really only need a ball with a high rating if you plan to lift weights on top of it, or if you're going to use it in a place where punctures are likely, such as your backyard. If you do get a puncture, it's best to buy a new ball—a repaired hole is a dangerous weak spot.

Inflating your ball

Many balls come with a special pump. If yours doesn't, you can either buy the tool separately, use a mattress pump, or take it to a gas station and use the air pump there. Inflate your ball only to the recommended diameter, which is printed on the ball and on the box. Don't inflate it any larger than this.

If you are a beginner and find the rolling motion very unsettling, you can deflate your ball slightly, which will prevent it rolling as much. However, once you are more familiar with the equipment, try reinflating it to its full size, as this will challenge and improve your coordination.

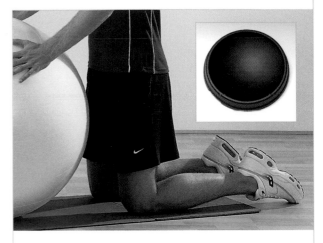

Ball size guide

Your height	Ball size	
4ft 11in to 5ft 4in	21in (53cm)	
5ft 5in to 5ft 11in	25in (65cm)	
6ft or taller	29in (75cm)	

What else you will need

- A well-ventilated room, with space to move and a clean floor, free of sharp objects. If you want to stop the ball rolling as much, try exercising on a carpet or long grass.
- Comfortable clothes, in which you can move easily. Either go barefoot or wear good non-slip sneakers.
- Water, to prevent dehydration.
- An exercise mat, available in most sports stores, to protect your back and head on the floor.
- A stabilizer base, an optional extra that can help you get used to the movement of the ball (see picture above). Alternatively, place the ball against a solid wall.

Know Your Ball

Many fitness aids, like weights machines and abs cages, are used to stabilize your position and help keep your body in the correct alignment. The ball, however, does the opposite. Because it is an unstable piece of equipment and because it is up to you to keep your body in position, it's useful to spend some time getting used to the feel of the ball before you start the exercises. In exercises like the sitting balance (see pages 48–49) you could fall off if you're not careful, so take each new exercise slowly and try the basic positions on page 13 before your first workout—many of the exercises actually begin with one of these positions.

SAFETY FIRST

Always place both hands on the ball and sit, lean, or lower yourself onto it slowly. It can easily roll away, leaving you to fall flat on the floor. For your first few workouts, you might want to get used to the rolling motion by resting the ball against a sturdy wall or using a special ball stabilizer, available at most sporting goods stores.

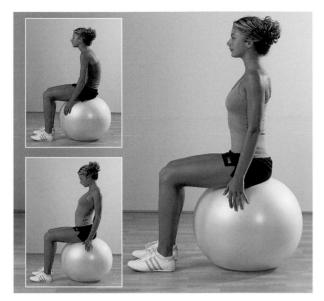
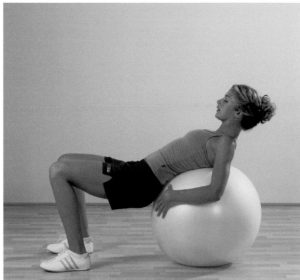
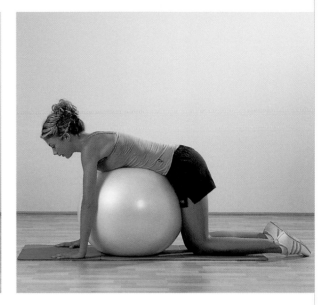

Basic sit

Stand with your back to the ball. Use your hands to steady the ball and sit down on top of it. Place your feet flat on the floor about shoulder-width apart. If the ball is the correct height, your thighs should be parallel to the floor and at right angles to your knees. Straighten your back and push the top of your head toward the ceiling. Relax your shoulders, lengthen your neck and drop your chin slightly so the back of your neck is straight and long.

Many people sit with a jutting chin, slumped shoulders, and a curved lower back; other people let their buttocks stick out and their stomach sag forward (see insets). Not only are these postures unattractive, but they can also weaken your back muscles and cause tension and pain.

Tighten your abdominals and roll the ball forward and back until your hips are directly under your shoulders. Your lower back should be neither very rounded nor very arched. This is known as neutral alignment. Keep it in mind not only when exercising on the ball but also in everyday life.

Basic lie

From the basic sit position you can move into the next key position. Slowly walk your feet forward and lie back on the ball. Allow the ball to roll until it is under your lower back, the back of your rib cage, and your shoulders. Keep your abdominals tight and your hips lifted. From here you can drop your shoulders and head back into the start position of the basic ab curl (see pages 40–41), but even holding this position works your abdominals.

All-fours

Kneel with the ball in front of you. Pull the ball in close and wrap your upper body up and over the ball. If the ball is the correct size, you should be able to place your hands on the floor in front of the ball and keep your knees on the floor. Check that your weight is equally distributed between your hands and knees. Tighten your abdominals. This is the start position for exercises such as the superman (see pages 26–27) and the ab contraction (see pages 42–43), but is also a good way of stretching your upper back (see pages 70–71).

Getting out of the positions

When coming out of positions, you need to make yourself as stable as possible. Place your feet or hands on the floor in what seems like the most comfortable position. If you are sitting or lying back on the ball, place both feet on the floor quite wide apart. Roll your buttocks toward your feet and lower slowly to the floor. If you are in a prone position with your hands on the floor and your legs on the ball, place one foot in front of the ball or lower your knees to the floor. When you're ready, use your hands to help you stand. If your head has been lower than your heart, bring it up slowly to give the blood a chance to drain from your head.

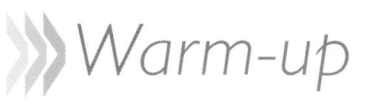

Warm-up

No matter how fit or flexible you are, the warm-up is an essential part of every workout. It gives your body and mind a chance to prepare for exercise. Your warm-up doesn't have to take long and isn't difficult. It is, however, crucial if you want to get the most out of exercise and avoid injury—never be tempted to skip it.

Performing even the simplest of toning or stretching moves when your muscles are cold puts you at risk for injury. A good warm-up consists of gentle exercise that is within your normal range of movement and that gets your heart pumping faster and more blood flowing to your muscles. It also generates heat, loosening your joints and muscles and enabling them to stretch further and more safely.

One way to warm up is to do 5 to 10 minutes of cardiovascular exercise, such as gentle walking, jogging, cycling, or stair-climbing. But you may find it more fun to perform some mobilization exercises with the ball. Learn the following sequence by heart, so you can go from one exercise to the next without stopping. Put on some lively music, and get your heart pumping.

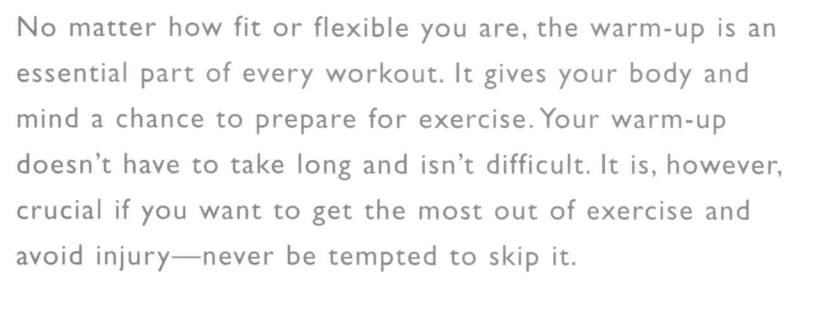

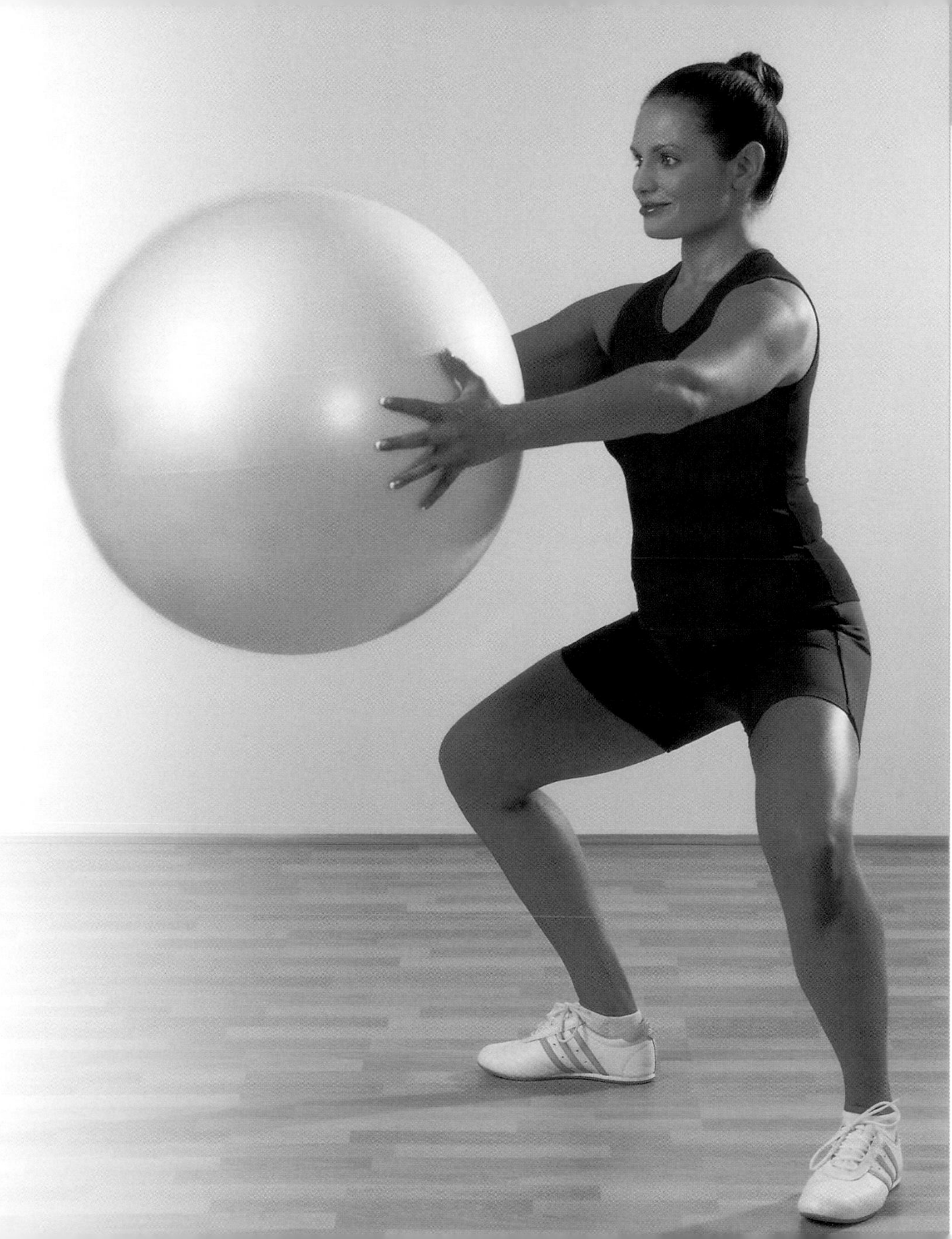

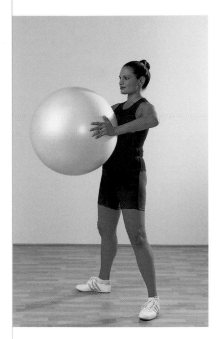
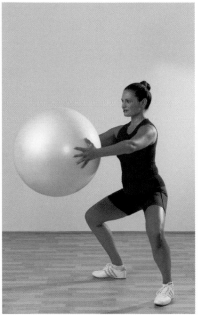
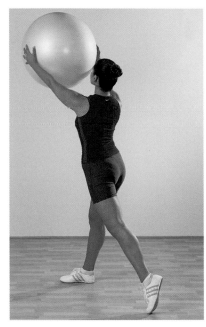

Push and swing

1 Stand with your feet wider than shoulder-width apart and turned out slightly—don't lock your knees. Hold the ball with both hands in front of your chest.

2 Slowly bend your knees and push your buttocks back and down—don't let your knees go past your toes. At the same time, straighten your arms and push the ball out in front of you. Hold for a second, then slowly straighten your legs and return to the start position. Repeat 10 to 12 times.

3 Hold the ball in front of your hips—don't lock your elbows. Twist your body to the right, moving from your hips, and transfer your weight to your right leg. At the same time, swing the ball as far as you can up and back to the right. Immediately return the ball to center and swing it to the left. Do 10 to 12 swings on each side in a constant, controlled movement.

Ball twist

1 Stand with your legs wide apart, knees bent slightly, and your feet pointing out. Hold the ball in front of you, level with your chest. Your arms should be straight, but don't lock your elbows. Twist your shoulders and the ball to the left as far as you can, but keep your hips facing forward. Return to center, then twist to the right. Do 10 to 15 twists to each side.

2 Repeat step 1, but each time you twist to the side, bend from your waist and touch the ball on the floor behind your leg. Do 10 to 15 twists and bends on each side.

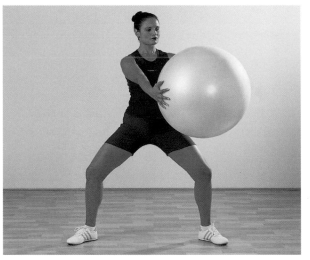
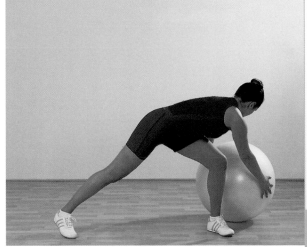

≫ Warm-up (2)

As you're warming up, prepare your mind for exercise. Practice moving smoothly and with control. Read these technique pointers and keep them in mind throughout your exercise session.

Technique dos and don'ts

- Do keep your abdominals tight throughout the exercises. You don't need to suck your stomach right in, but pull your belly button in toward your spine to protect your back.
- Don't lock your joints. You could risk overstretching or jarring them. If you have to straighten your arms or legs as part of an exercise, your elbows or knees should remain slightly bent.
- Do keep your shoulders and neck relaxed. Tilt your chin slightly toward your chest so your neck is in line with your spine. If you have to place your hands on your head, support the weight of your head lightly with your fingertips—don't pull on your neck.
- Don't let your knees go past your toes. If you have to bend your legs in a standing position, like the wall squat (see pages 58–59), look down at your knees to check they aren't farther forward than your toes.
- Do breathe out through your mouth during the most difficult part of the exercise, such as the upward crunch in the basic ab curl (see pages 40–41). Breathe in through your nose during the less difficult part of the exercise—as you are lowering your body back down, for instance.
- Don't overstretch or bounce a stretch. Stretch slowly and steadily to the point where it becomes uncomfortable, but not painful.
- Do take regular sips of water, particularly if you are feeling hot or perspiring a lot.
- Do take each exercise slowly. Stop and rest if you really can't do any more or if you start to shake.

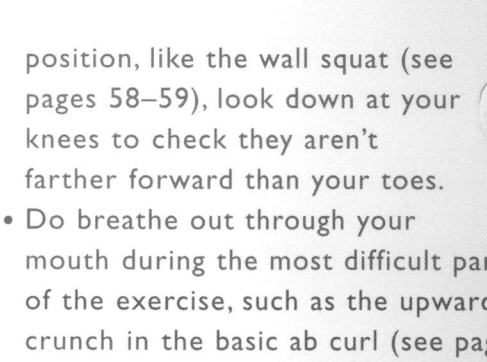

Leg catch

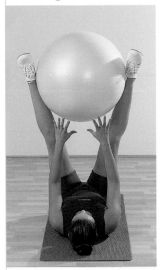

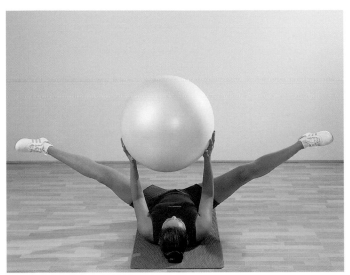

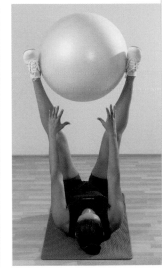

1 Lie on your back on a mat. Straighten your legs so the soles of your feet point to the ceiling. Place the ball between your ankles. Raise your hands toward the ball.

2 Quickly open your legs out wide and catch the ball with both hands.

3 Use your hands to throw the ball back into the air.

4 Catch the ball between your ankles. Repeat 10 times.

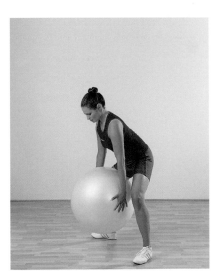

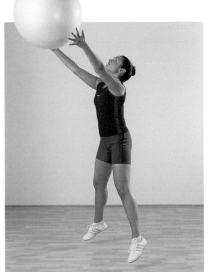

Swing jump

1 Stand with your legs wider than shoulder-width apart and your knees bent. Hold the ball in both hands and bend forward from your waist so the ball is between your legs.

2 Bend your knees and jump. At the same time, swing your arms forward and up to throw the ball in the air. Catch the ball and bend your knees as you land. Repeat 8 times.

⟩⟩ *Cool-down*

If you exercise regularly at the gym or in a class, you might be used to doing stretches during your cool-down. However, stretches are included in all the routines in this book, so a cool-down after your ball workout is more about preparing your body for the rest of the day. Psychologically, it's great to reflect on the activity you've just done and how much better you feel for doing it. It gives your mind a break from the constant flow of thoughts we have in our daily lives. The cool-down becomes even more important the busier our lives get: we're usually rushing about so much that we rarely make time to relax and unwind. Enjoy the following cool-down positions.

The leg elevation position (see below) will relax your body and give your heartbeat a chance to return to normal. It's particularly good if you sit or stand for long periods during the day, which can cause the blood to pool in your lower legs. Elevating your legs relieves the pressure on the veins and muscles that return the blood up to your heart. In contrast, the tip-up position is a fun challenge to improve your balance. It gets the blood flowing to your head and really wakes you up again for the rest of the day.

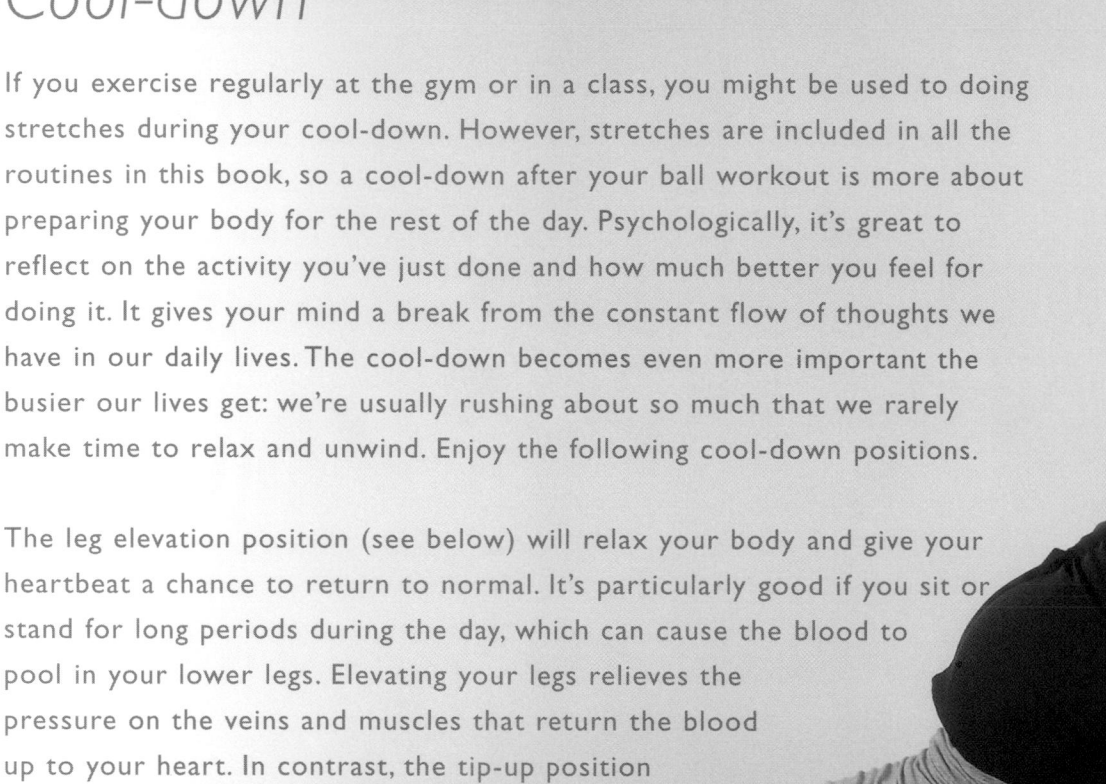

Leg elevation

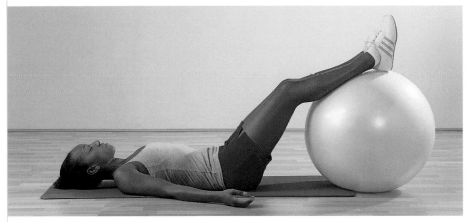

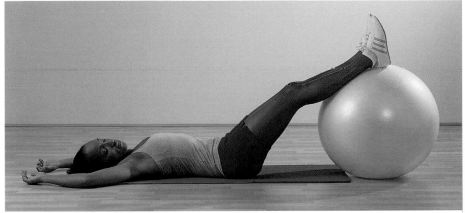

1 Lie on your back on a mat. Rest your calves and ankles on top of the ball. Your knees may fall apart a little—adjust your legs until you feel comfortable. Lay your arms by your sides, palms facing up and fingers loosely curled. Close your eyes.

2 If you feel more comfortable, you can rest your arms on the floor behind your head. Relax your whole body from the tips of your toes to your shoulders, jaw, and face. Let your hips and rib cage sink lower into the floor, and feel the tension leave your neck. Notice any minute changes taking place in your body. Don't think about what it is—just notice it. If you mind slips into thinking about the tasks you must do later or the work you have to do tomorrow, draw it back to focus on your body. Stay like this for a few minutes.

Tip-up

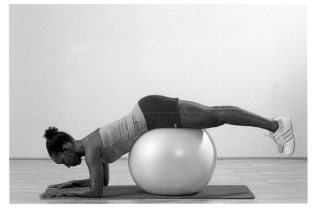

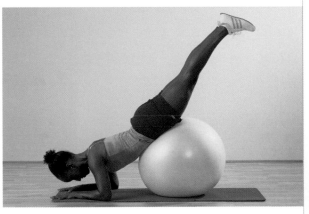

1 Kneel with the ball in front of you. Roll forward onto the ball until it is under your hips and you can rest your hands and forearms on the floor. Raise your legs.

2 Tighten your abdominals. Gradually move your body weight forward and lift your straightened legs in the air as high as you can. Hold for 10 seconds. Return your feet to the floor, rest for 10 seconds, then repeat. You may find this move difficult at first; work it slowly and aim to get your legs a little higher with each workout.

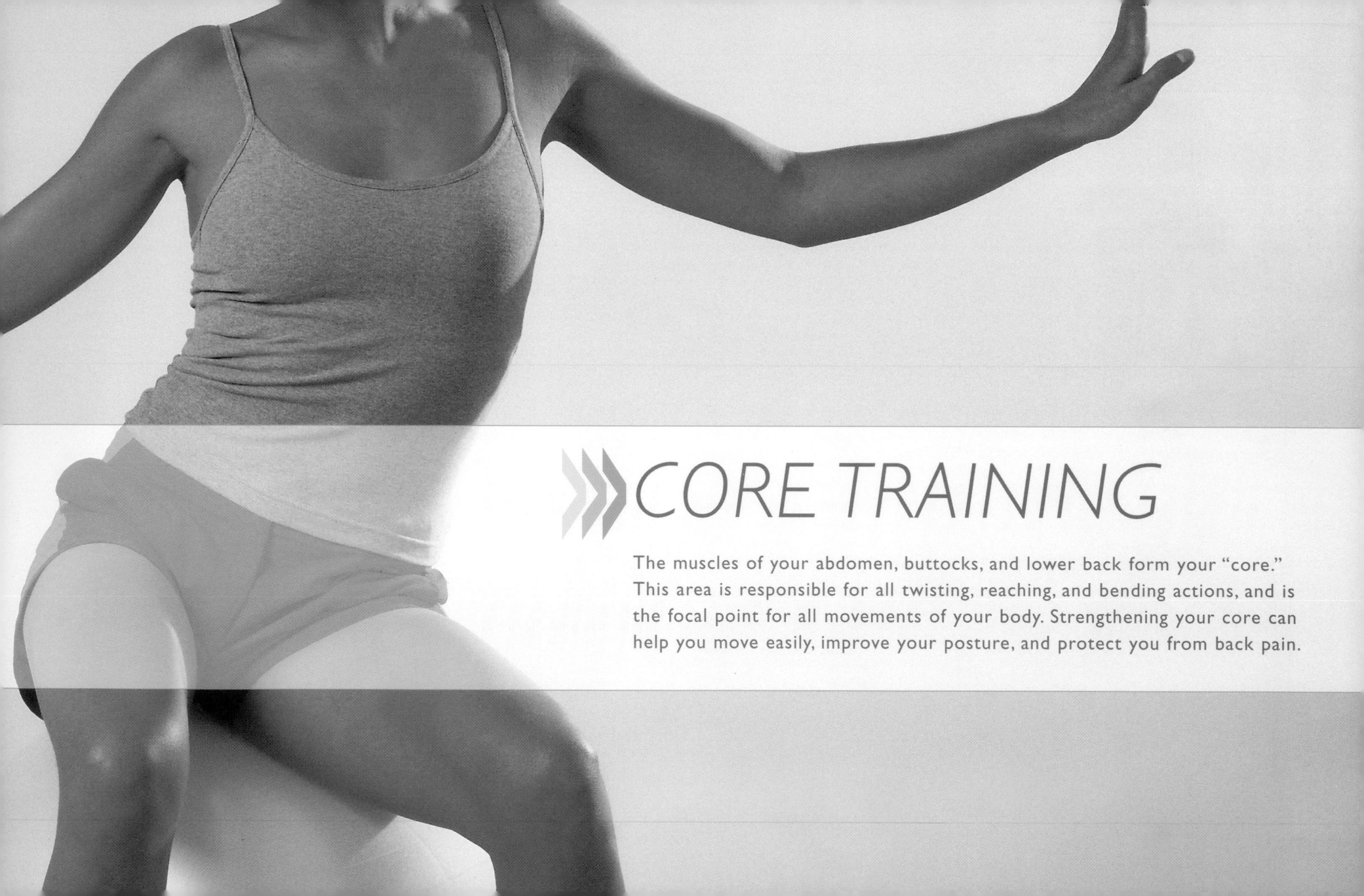

>>CORE TRAINING

The muscles of your abdomen, buttocks, and lower back form your "core." This area is responsible for all twisting, reaching, and bending actions, and is the focal point for all movements of your body. Strengthening your core can help you move easily, improve your posture, and protect you from back pain.

Strong core muscles are important at all times and at all stages of life: they enable you to sit upright at a desk or perform better at many sports; they give you the strength to lift your kids; and they can help you stay active and independent in later life. If you allow your core to become weak, not only will you look out of shape, but pretty soon you'll start to feel it. Weak abdominals can lead to a sagging stomach, which can be pulled even more out of shape if you overeat. And one of the major causes of back pain is lack of strength in the torso area. Because we stand upright—unlike our fellow mammals—the weight of our heads and upper bodies places pressure on our lower backs. This pressure increases with poor posture—if you lean back and let your stomach protrude. Strong core muscles will help pull your body upright and take some of the weight off the joints in your spine.

SAFETY FIRST

Many of the core training moves are isometric, which means that you are using your muscles to hold a position rather than to power a move. You need to keep breathing throughout the exercise to supply your muscles with oxygen—if you don't, they will quickly become exhausted.

To have a strong, stress-free core, you need to work both the front and back of your torso. The main muscles here are:

- The rectus abdominus, which runs vertically from your lower chest to your pubic bone. This muscle is the one that shows as a "six pack" on some men. It helps bend your body forward and keeps your spine still when you lift a heavy weight off the floor.
- The internal and external obliques, which wrap around the sides of your torso. They help the rectus abdominus bend the body forward and enable you to twist and to bend to the sides.
- The transverse abdominus, which lies underneath the rectus abdominus and runs horizontally across the stomach. It isn't involved in much movement, but you can feel it when you cough or sneeze.
- The lower-back muscles, in particular the erector spinae, which lie on either side of your spine. These muscles help bend your spine

backward and work with the abdominals to stabilize your spine when you make other movements.

Ways to work your program
The exercises in this section will build your confidence on the ball and will help you better perform other exercises. Include one or two core-training exercises at the start of each session to work these key muscles. This will also remind you to focus on your midsection in all the following exercises and to keep good posture when not exercising.

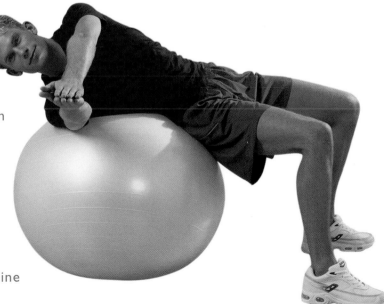

The Seated Roll

When you sit on the ball, you are on an unstable base. This means your abdominal muscles and all the small muscles along the length of your spine have to work hard and make constant, small readjustments in order to maintain a balanced, upright position. You can even use an exercise ball in place of a chair—while at work, for example—in order to stimulate your core muscles throughout the day.

The Seated Roll exercises consist of very small movements originating from your pelvis, stomach, back, and sides. The ball exaggerates these movements as it rolls beneath you, helping you to target the correct muscles.

Keep your stomach pulled in and feel the benefits from each stage of the exercise.

Tilting and circling your hips and pelvis is great for the obliques and the rectus abdominus.

As you raise your hips, concentrate on squeezing each side of your waist.

BALL CHAIR: A stability ball chair encourages "active sitting," which is when you subconsciously adjust your posture in order to maintain balance. Sitting on a ball chair for a few hours a day can improve balance and tone your core muscles. Some studies suggest that it may also improve your concentration.

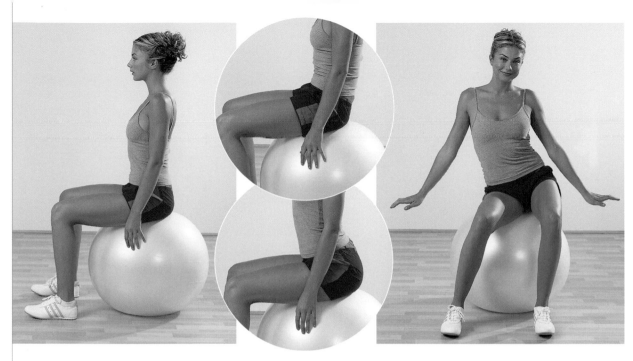
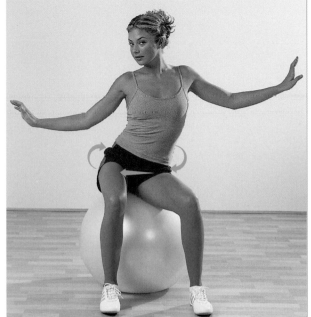

1 Sit upright on the ball with your feet about shoulder-width apart and your knees at right angles. Drop your chin slightly and raise the top of your head toward the ceiling. Tighten your abdominals and straighten your back. Your pelvis and hips should be directly under your ribs and shoulders. Remember this position: your pelvis is now in "neutral" alignment (see also page 13).

2 Keep your upper body still. Further contract your stomach muscles so your pelvis tucks under and your hips tilt forward. The ball will roll to accommodate this movement. Keep squeezing your stomach muscles and hold for a count of two.

Lengthen your abdominals and contract your lower-back muscles to tilt your pelvis back. The ball will roll backward, too. Hold for a count of two. Tilt your pelvis forward and back a few times and note how far the ball rolls in each direction. This shows you the full range of movement in your pelvis.

3 Return to the neutral position of step 1. Keep your upper body and legs still and your hips facing forward, but contract the left side of your torso to raise your left hip. Allow the ball to roll beneath you. Return to center, then repeat on the right-hand side. Tilt your hips from one side to the other a few times. Note how far the ball rolls in each direction. Over the weeks, you should see improvements in your hip mobility.

4 Finally, keep your upper body and feet in place and rotate your hips, both clockwise and counter-clockwise. This works your waist as you manipulate your hips and the ball in a full circle. Move smoothly and repeat a few times in each direction.

Upper-body Rotation

This exercise focuses mainly on the obliques at the sides of your abdomen, which help twist your torso. Toning these muscles is essential if you want a trim waist and a strong midsection, improving spinal mobility as it loosens the often-neglected ligaments and joints of your lower back.

The upper-body rotation helps build total core strength, since you need to keep your lower body still and lifted as you twist your arms and upper body to the side. You'll notice this particularly in step 3, when the ball supports less of your body weight and you have to work hard to stay horizontal. Focus on moving steadily throughout the exercise.

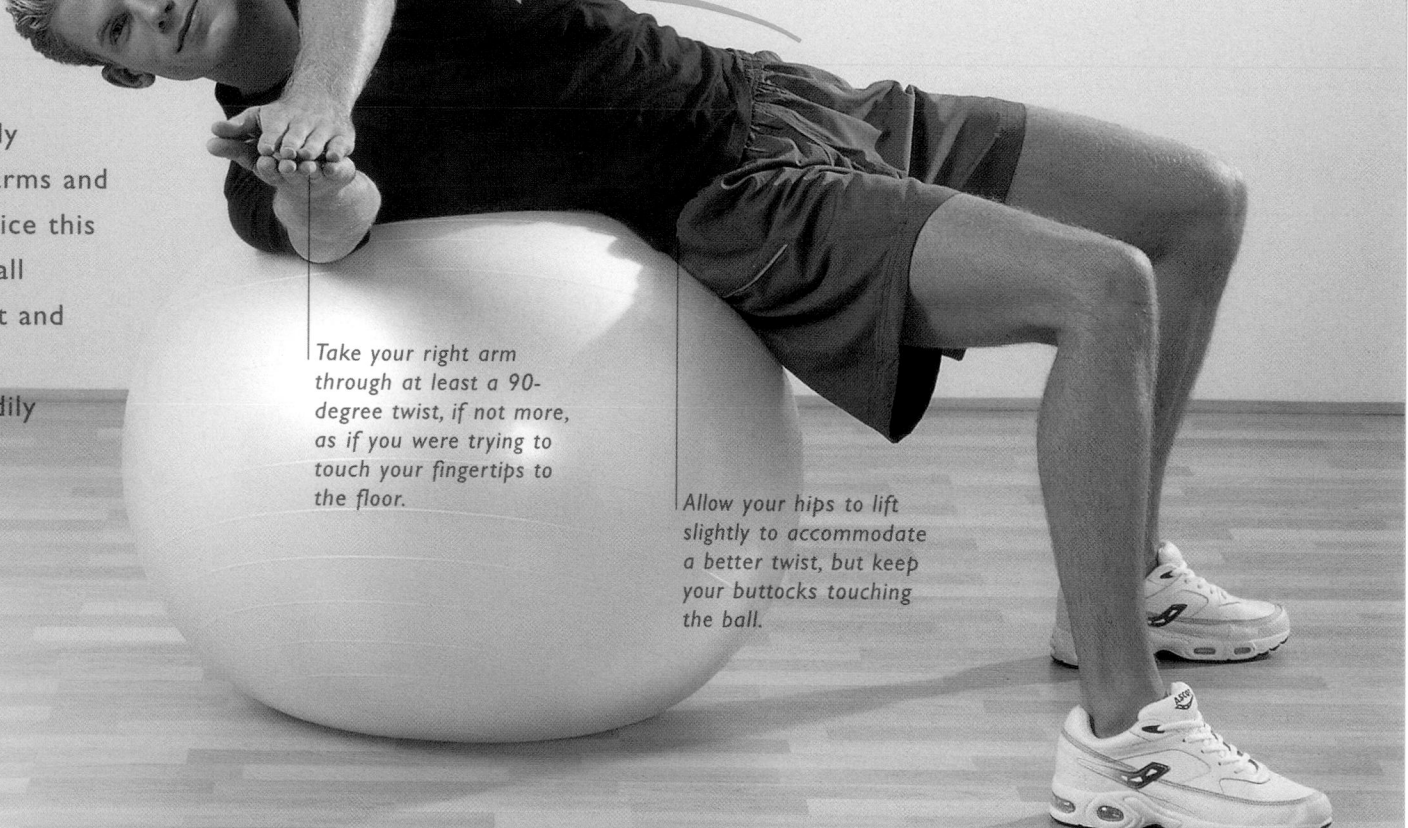

Concentrate on keeping your core solid. Move your upper body around this point.

Take your right arm through at least a 90-degree twist, if not more, as if you were trying to touch your fingertips to the floor.

Allow your hips to lift slightly to accommodate a better twist, but keep your buttocks touching the ball.

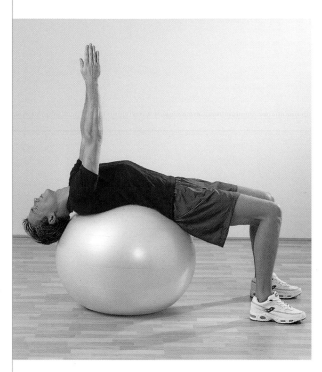

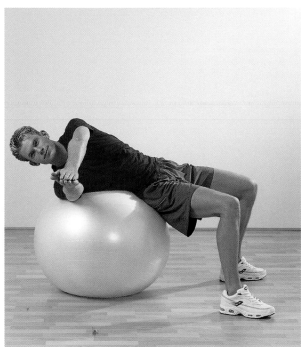

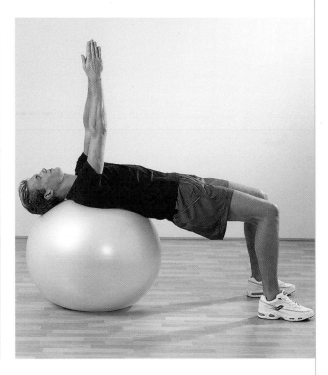

1 Sit upright on the ball with your feet on the floor. Walk your feet forward and lie back. Relax your head and shoulders until the ball is supporting the whole of your back. Reach both arms toward the ceiling and press your palms together.

2 Keep your knees still and your buttocks raised. Lift your head. Lower both arms to your right for the count of three. The ball will roll slightly to the left. Let your left hip rise a little, if necessary, but not too much. Keep both arms straight with the palms pressed together. Slowly return to center for a count of three. Lower to the other side. Repeat 8 times on each side. Rest for 30 seconds, then move on to step 3.

3 Return your arms to center. Walk your feet farther forward until just your upper back, shoulders, neck, and head are on the ball. Pull in your buttocks and abdominals so your hips are level with your knees. Reach your arms up, palms pressed together. Twist to each side as before. Repeat 8 times on each side.

Easy alternative

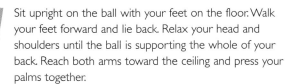

If you find it difficult to stay balanced, try this move on the floor. Lie down on a mat with your knees bent and feet flat on the floor. Reach both arms toward the ceiling and press your palms together. Twist to each side as above.

❯❯ Superman

This exercise works the erector spinae, which run along either side of your spine. You will feel tiny muscular adjustments here as you try to find the correct position. It is a challenging move and you may find it difficult to balance at first. Pulling in your abdominals will help. It may take you a few attempts to lift both arms off the floor. If you can't do it at first, persevere with step 1 for three to four workouts, then try again.

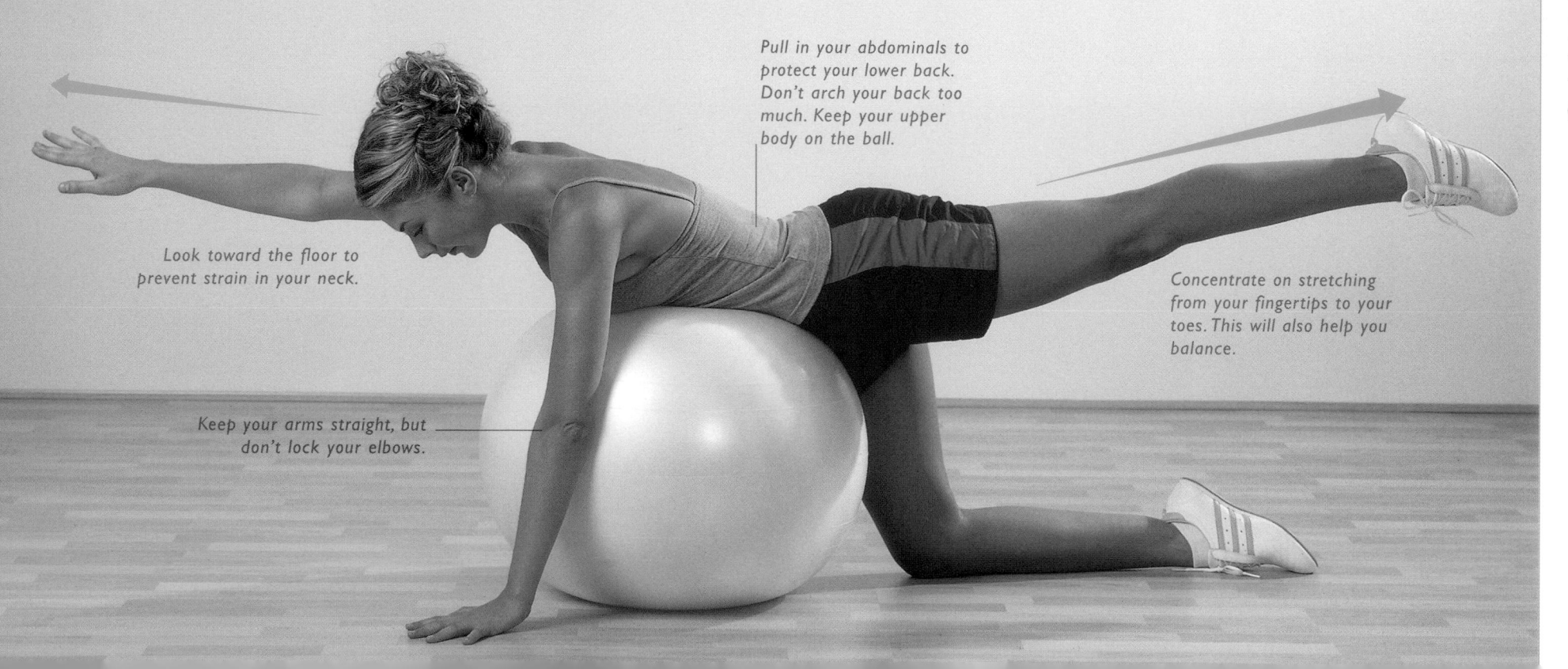

Pull in your abdominals to protect your lower back. Don't arch your back too much. Keep your upper body on the ball.

Look toward the floor to prevent strain in your neck.

Concentrate on stretching from your fingertips to your toes. This will also help you balance.

Keep your arms straight, but don't lock your elbows.

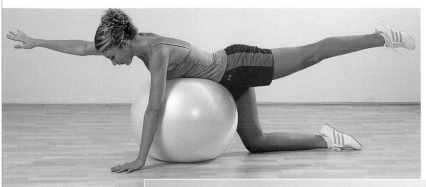

1 Kneel with the ball in front of you. Keep your knees on the floor as you roll your torso up and onto the ball. Place your hands on the floor in front of the ball about shoulder-width apart. Next, lift your right arm out straight in front of you. At the same time, lift your left leg out straight behind you and point your toes. Move slowly as you find your balance. Keep both hips and your left knee pointing toward the floor. Hold for 20 seconds. Keep breathing.

2 If you feel balanced, stretch your left arm in front of you as well. Try to keep your body flat, but, if necessary, you can raise your left leg slightly to help you balance. Don't twist your hips; keep them facing downward. Hold for 20 seconds, or as long as possible.

3 Place both hands on the floor. Lean into the ball. Lift your left leg up behind you as high as you can. Allow your left hip to come off the ball. Hold for 20 seconds. Lower your leg. Repeat steps 1 to 3 on your right leg.

Beyond the basics

This is a fun alternative that will improve your balance and work your lower back. Begin with your hips on the ball, arms and legs straight, hands and toes on the floor. Find a point of balance, then quickly lift your arms and legs high behind you. Hold for as long as possible. When you start to fall, replace your hands and feet on the floor.

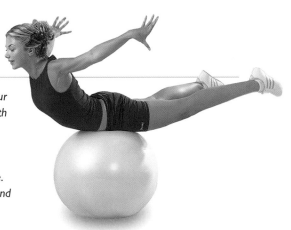

⟩⟩ *Push-up Perfecter*

This is an isometric exercise (see page 21) that uses your core muscles, particularly your transverse abdominals, to keep you steady on top of the ball and to keep your midsection lifted. When you're holding the position, it doesn't look like you're doing much, but it is a highly effective exercise—you'll feel this particularly in the last two steps.

This is a great exercise for improving posture, helping prevent the arched back and sagging stomach that can make you look less toned than you are.

SAFETY FIRST

If you have weak stomach muscles or suffer from lower-back pain, stick with the easiest position at first (step 1). If you feel strong enough after six workouts including this move try step 2. Progress to step 3 in the same way. If you feel any pain, stop immediately and seek medical advice.

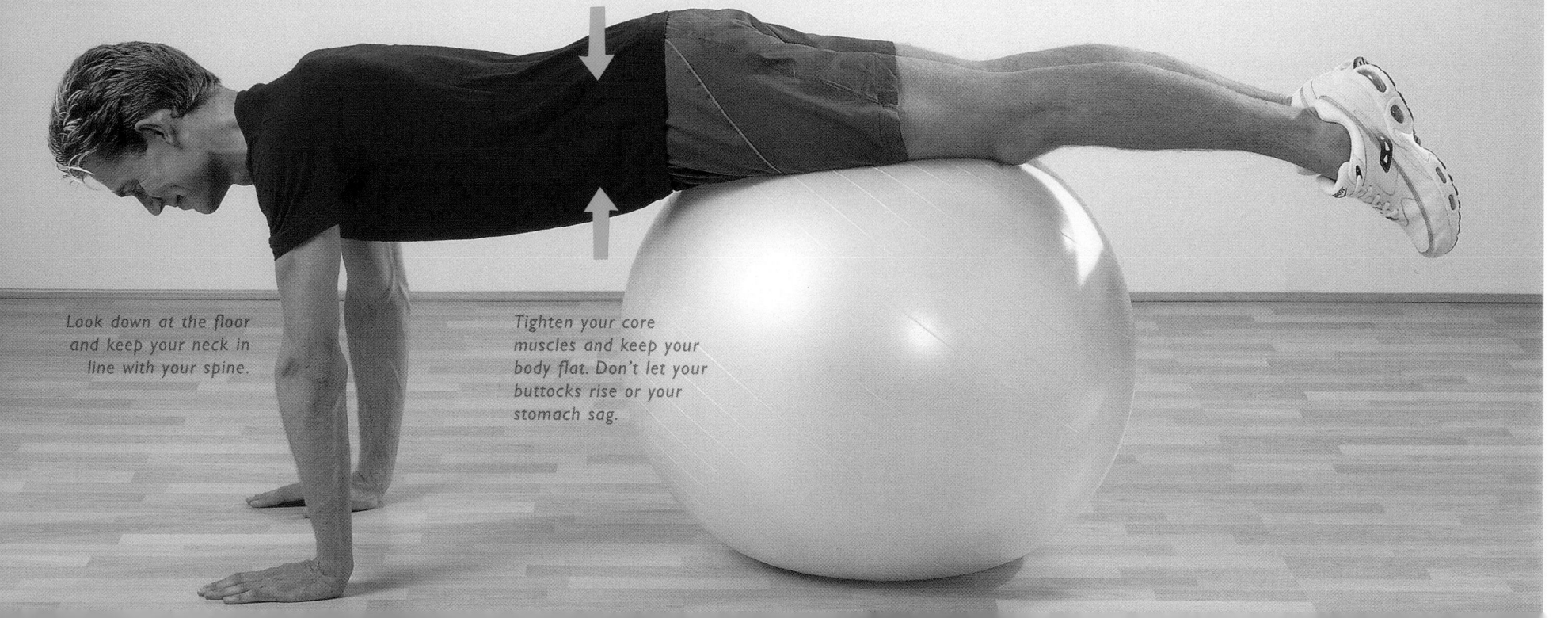

Look down at the floor and keep your neck in line with your spine.

Tighten your core muscles and keep your body flat. Don't let your buttocks rise or your stomach sag.

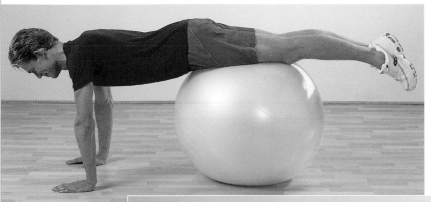

1 Kneel with the ball in front of you. Keep your knees on the floor and roll your torso up and onto the ball. Place your hands on the floor in front of the ball, about shoulder-width apart. Take your body weight on your hands and walk them forward until your hips and thighs are on top of the ball. At the same time lift your feet and legs. Your legs should be slightly apart. Breathe as you hold for 10 seconds.

2 Slowly walk your hands farther forward until your knees are on top of the ball. Don't let your feet and legs rise or your back or stomach sag; concentrate on keeping your body in a straight line. Breathe as you hold for 10 seconds.

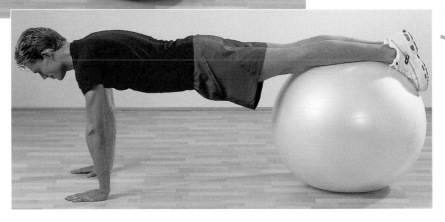

3 Slowly walk your hands farther forward until your shins and ankles are on top of the ball. Breathe as you hold for 10 seconds.

Perfect partner

This is good preparation for the more challenging push-up (see pages 34–35). Practice steps 2 and 3 of the push-up perfecter before you do the beyond the basics version of the push-up.

❯❯ The Plank

This difficult position recruits all the muscles of your torso, but particularly your transverse abdominals, which are deep and run horizontally across the stomach. The plank works your muscles isometrically, meaning that they become stronger and more toned by holding a position rather than by repeated movements, such as sit-ups. In this case your abdominals have to stabilize your position, prevent the ball from rolling, and keep almost all your body weight suspended. Until you get used to the correct position, you may find it helpful to do this exercise in front of a mirror so you can check that your body remains in a straight line throughout. As you get stronger over the weeks, hold the position for longer each time.

Squeeze your buttocks, abdominals, and the muscles of your lower back. Don't allow your buttocks to rise or your stomach to sag.

You will feel your arms working to support your weight. Keep them at 90 degrees to the floor.

Concentrate on lengthening your body from your ankles to your shoulders.

SAFETY FIRST

If your muscles start to weaken or tremble, or if you feel you're about to lose your balance, lower your knees to the floor, rest for 20 seconds, then begin again.

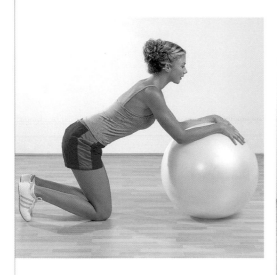

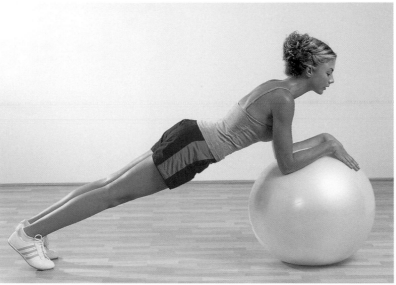

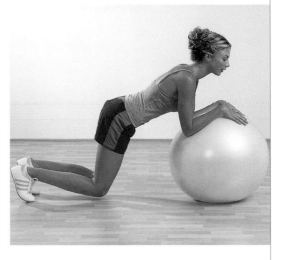

1 Kneel with the ball an arm's length in front of you. Tighten your abdominals. Lean forward and rest your hands and forearms on top of the ball. Curl your toes under and rest them on the floor. Look at a point on the floor just beyond the ball.

2 Lift your knees and straighten your legs. Allow the ball to roll forward as you adjust your buttocks and torso until your body forms a straight line from the backs of your ankles to the back of your neck. Hold for 10 seconds. Keep your neck in line with your spine. Keep breathing throughout.

3 To come out of this position, bend your knees slowly and place them on the floor. Then roll back to kneeling.

● **REST AND REPEAT**
Rest for: 20 seconds
Repeat: twice more, resting in between

Beyond the basics

In this alternative your body is farther away from the ball so your arms and abdominals have to work harder to keep the ball still and your body in a straight line. Stand with the ball about an arm's length in front of you. Tighten your abdominals. Bend forward and place your hands on top of the ball. Your arms should be straight, but don't lock your elbows. Walk your legs behind you until your body forms a straight line from the backs of your ankles to the back of your neck. Hold for 5 seconds. Breathe throughout. Repeat twice more.

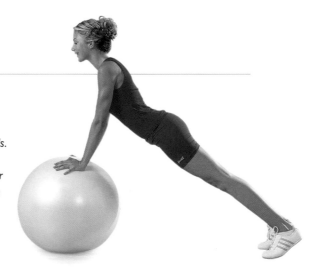

THE PLANK

31

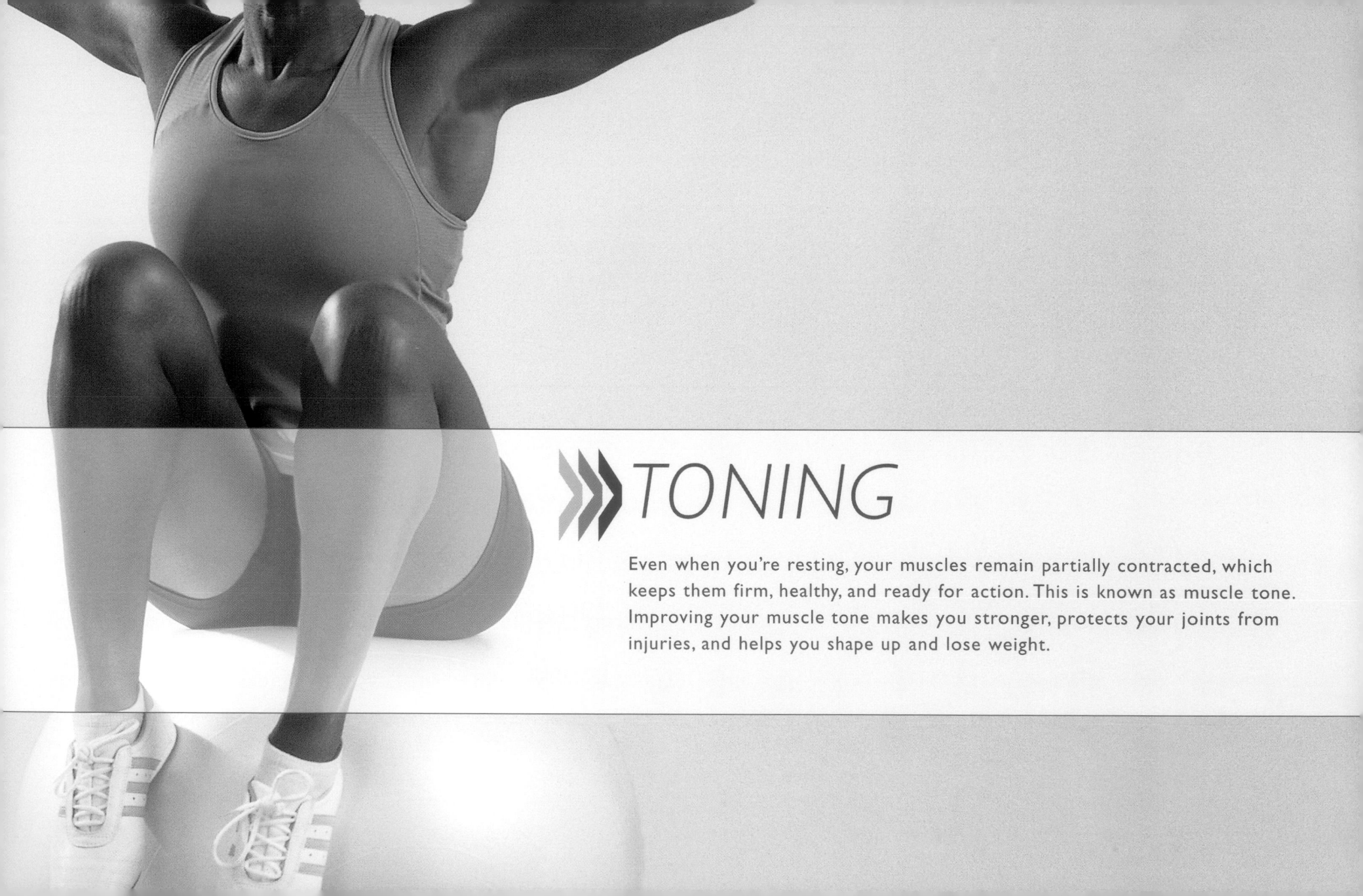

>>TONING

Even when you're resting, your muscles remain partially contracted, which keeps them firm, healthy, and ready for action. This is known as muscle tone. Improving your muscle tone makes you stronger, protects your joints from injuries, and helps you shape up and lose weight.

Muscles work by contraction. In order to bend your arm, for example, the biceps muscle in your upper arm contracts, pulling your lower arm up toward your shoulder. To make your muscles stronger and more defined, you need to give them something to contract against. To strengthen the biceps, you could hold a dumbbell in your hand to add resistance. All toning exercises involve using some sort of resistance, whether it's in the form of extra weights, such as dumbbells or barbells; specially designed resistance tools, such as rubberized dynaband straps; or gravity and your own body weight, for exercises like chin-ups and push-ups.

Toning on the exercise ball generally uses your own body weight as resistance. But an exercise ball adds a new dimension to toning, as it allows you to manipulate your

body in many different ways. So not only can you work on your own with the minimum of equipment, but you also have the variety and flexibility of moves you would normally get from a whole array of equipment. Even a small change of position on the ball can increase or decrease the intensity of the exercise, meaning you can perform several versions of the exercise in quick succession, with only short breaks in between. This ensures you get a maximum intensity workout in a short amount of time. Moreover, the ball offers a safe support, so you stay balanced and in the correct stance—when performing the wall squat (see pages 58–59) or the butt kick (see pages 50–51), for example. And this, in turn, allows you to get the most out of your exercise.

Ways to work your program

After performing a few toning exercises in a row, you may feel your muscles begin to tire and ache. If this happens, perform some of the stretching moves between the toning exercises to allow your muscles to recover.

Alternatively, work through all of the toning exercises and then do some, or all, of the stretches afterwards.

To judge your progress, aim to get through the complete range of toning exercises a minimum of twice a week for six consecutive weeks. At that stage you should notice significant improvements in muscle tone, as well as in your balance and posture. If you're short on time, use either a 15- or 30-minute routine (see pages 90–93) to pack a fast, efficient workout into even the busiest of days.

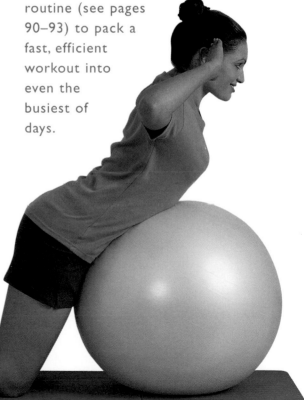

▶▶Push-up

This is a great all-around exercise. Raising and lowering the weight of your upper body tones the pectoral muscles of your chest, as well as your shoulders and triceps. And when you do a push-up on the ball, you also need to engage your abdominals and buttock muscles in order to keep your body steady and in alignment. This means you give your whole body a workout with just one exercise. The ball can be positioned in different ways depending on your level of fitness. In the basic position you feel the work mainly in your chest and arms. This exercise may not feel difficult, but it's good preparation for the more challenging version (see beyond the basics, page 35). This variation places an increased load on your abdominals, as your midsection muscles have to work really hard to keep your body rigid.

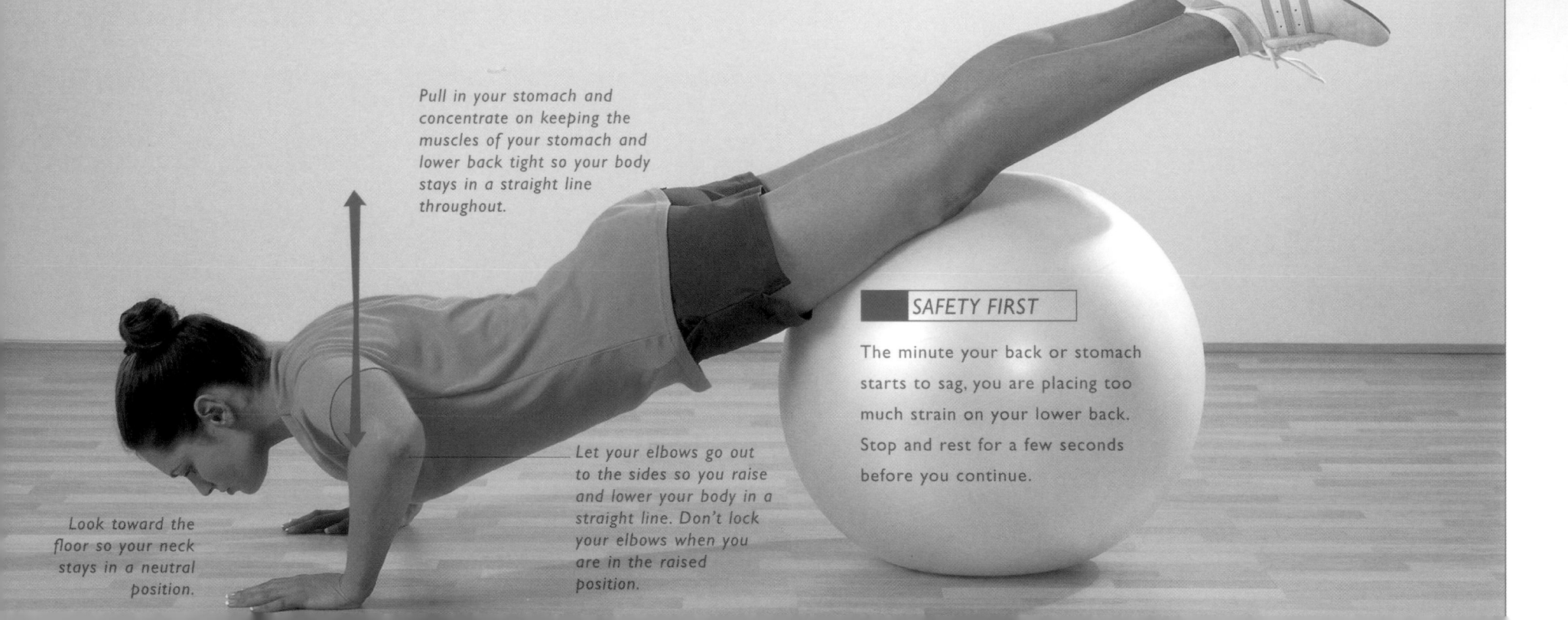

Pull in your stomach and concentrate on keeping the muscles of your stomach and lower back tight so your body stays in a straight line throughout.

Look toward the floor so your neck stays in a neutral position.

Let your elbows go out to the sides so you raise and lower your body in a straight line. Don't lock your elbows when you are in the raised position.

SAFETY FIRST

The minute your back or stomach starts to sag, you are placing too much strain on your lower back. Stop and rest for a few seconds before you continue.

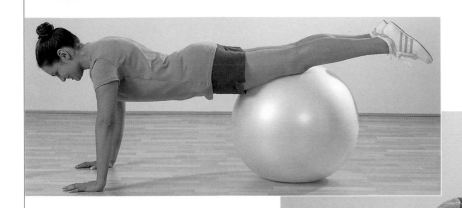

1 Kneel on the floor and place the ball in front of you. Roll your torso up onto the ball. Place your hands flat on the floor in front of you. Walk your hands forward until the ball is under your thighs, near your knees. Straighten your legs behind you so your body is horizontal. Your shoulders should be directly over your wrists.

2 Bend your arms and lower your chest for a count of two. Aim to get your nose close to the floor. Hold for a second, then straighten your arms for a count of two. Do 10–12 push-ups, breathing regularly throughout. Rest for 20 seconds, then move on to step 3.

3 Return to the starting position of step 1. Walk your hands slightly farther apart, just wider than shoulder-width. Lower half-way down for a count of two and hold for a count of two. Slowly straighten your arms. Keep breathing throughout. Repeat 10–12 times.

Beyond the basics

Walk your hands forward until your shins and ankles rest on the ball. Raise and lower your body in this position—it requires more work from your abdominals to keep your back straight and increases the load on your chest and arms, since less of your body weight is supported by the ball.

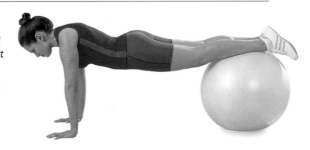

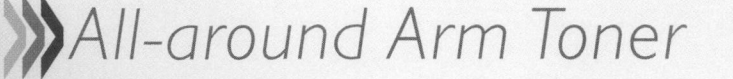

All-around Arm Toner

As we age, the muscles in our arms can sag. Unlike the biceps at the fronts of our arms—which are involved in many lifting actions—the triceps at the backs of our arms often need particular attention, because we rarely challenge them in daily life. Our shoulder muscles also benefit from strength exercises, because they protect the versatile shoulder joint and help move our arms in almost any direction.

This exercise works all the muscles in the arms and shoulders, giving them a toned and shapely appearance. This is usually difficult to achieve without weights, but you can use the ball to position your body so gravity adds resistance.

You may be tempted to hold your breath during these exercises because they involve only small movements, but you need to keep breathing regularly throughout to provide your muscles with oxygen and prevent cramps.

For the most benefit, work through the full range of movement in your arms and shoulders as you lift and lower.

Look down, but keep your head off the ball and don't tense your neck.

Tighten your abdominals to support your lower back and keep the ball in place.

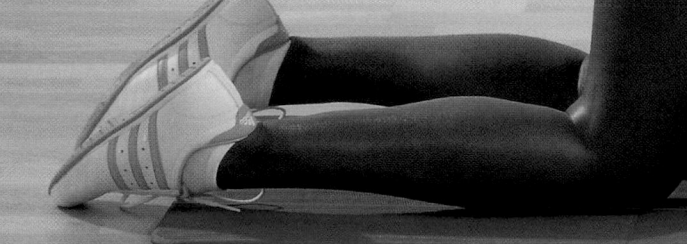

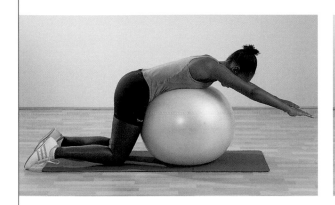

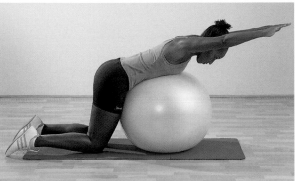

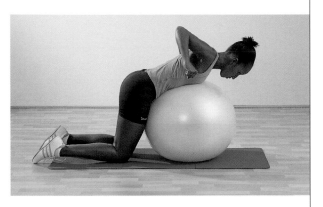

1 Kneel on the floor and place the ball in front of you. Lean forward over the ball so it is underneath your chest, rib cage, and stomach. Stretch your arms straight out in front of you, palms facing downward.

2 Lift your arms for a count of two, pressing them toward the ceiling. Hold for one count. Lower for a count of two. You should feel this in your shoulders. Repeat 16 times, rest for 30 seconds, then move on to step 3.

3 Return to step 1. Clench your hands into loose fists. Slowly pull your elbows up and back toward the ceiling. Move for a count of two. Hold for one count, then stretch them back out in front of you. You'll feel this in the middle of your upper back. Repeat 16 times, rest for 30 seconds, then move on to step 4.

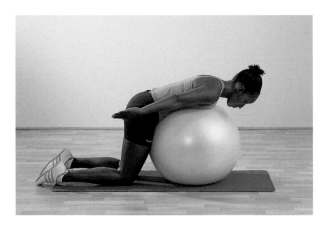

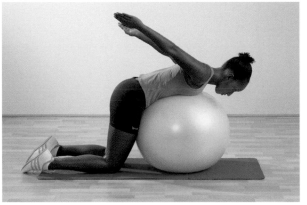

4 Return to the start position of step 1. Take both arms out straight behind you, with your wrists touching your hips and your palms facing upward.

5 Slowly raise your palms to the ceiling. Move for a count of two. Squeeze your shoulder blades together at the top. Lower, moving for a count of two. You'll see the benefits of this in the triceps at the backs of your upper arms. Repeat 16 times.

➤➤ *Back Toner*

Many people neglect to include back exercises in their workouts. But keeping your back muscles strong and flexible—along with your abdominals—is one of the best ways to keep your spine mobile and free of pain. This exercise mainly targets the muscles of your lower back, in particular the erector spinae, which support your spine and are the key to maintaining good posture. Pressing your arms back and up in step 3 also works the muscles in the center of your upper back, which pull your shoulder blades together and prevent slumped, rounded shoulders.

The closer the ball is to your body, the lower down your back you'll feel the effort. So if you want to focus on the base of your spine, start with the ball close to your hips. If you want to work the middle of your back, position the ball under your ribs and upper stomach.

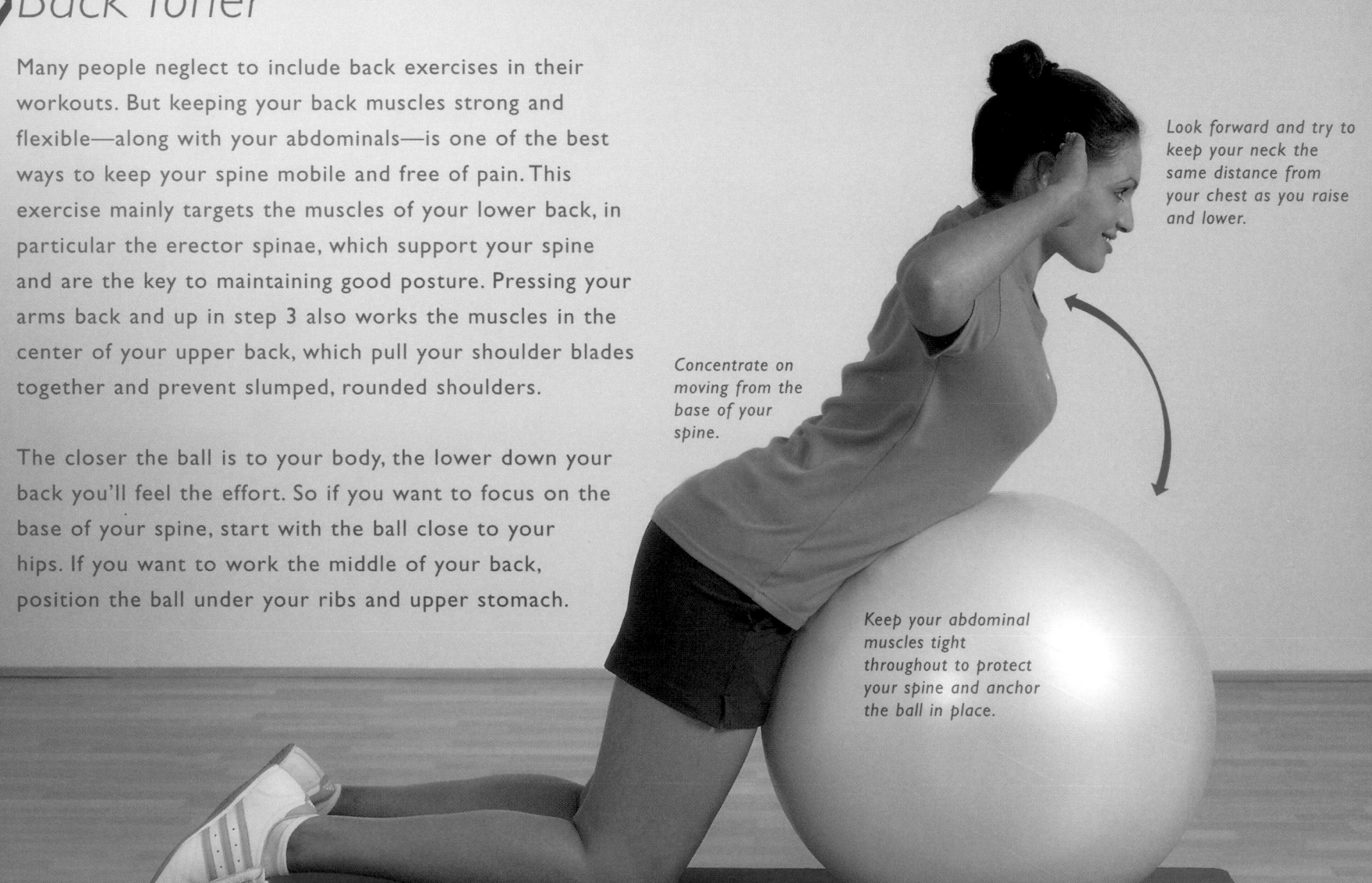

Look forward and try to keep your neck the same distance from your chest as you raise and lower.

Concentrate on moving from the base of your spine.

Keep your abdominal muscles tight throughout to protect your spine and anchor the ball in place.

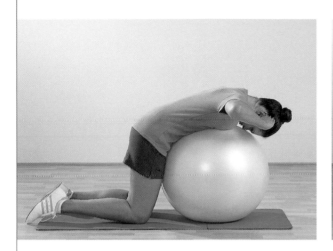

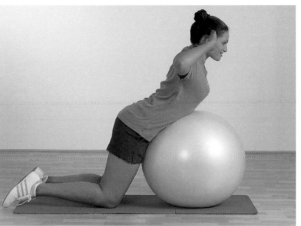

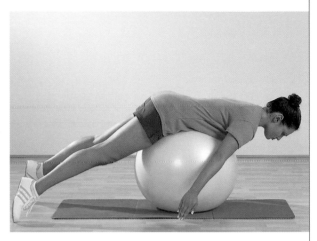

1 Kneel on the floor and place the ball in front of you. Relax your chest and rib cage onto the ball, but keep your knees firmly on the floor. Place your hands on either side of your head, with your elbows out to the sides and your fingertips resting behind your ears.

2 Lift your head and shoulders for a count of two, moving up and back off the ball. Hold for a count of two. Lower for a count of two. Keep breathing regularly throughout. Repeat 16 times, rest for 30 seconds, then move on to step 3.

3 Extend your legs straight behind you and rest on your toes, with your feet about shoulder-width apart. Roll forward slightly so the ball is under your hips Extend both arms out straight on either side of the ball, with your palms facing toward the ball and your fingertips close to the floor.

Beyond the basics

Begin in the start position of step 1, but extend both your arms in front of you so the insides of your arms touch your ears. As you arch back from this position, you have to lift your arms and, therefore, more body weight. Hold for a count of two, then lower for a count of two.

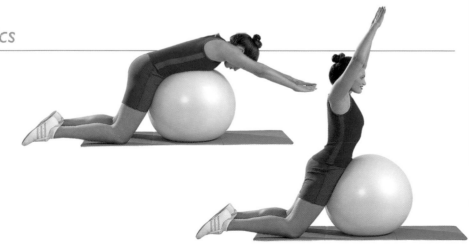

4 Lift your chest for a count of two. Simultaneously press both arms out to the sides and squeeze your shoulder blades together. Hold for a count of two. Lower for a count of two. Repeat 16 times.

Basic Ab Curl

The abdominals are one of the most important sets of muscles in the body. They protect important organs, and they're involved in all torso movement, from bending or twisting to jumping or standing up. Strengthening your abdominal muscles can help you achieve a flat stomach and can help support your spine and so prevent back pain. This exercise works the rectus abdominus, which runs down the front of your body, as well as the obliques at your sides.

Abdominal exercises performed on the floor have only limited effectiveness, because your range of movement is restricted. In contrast, the exercise ball allows you to place your body in a decline position (with your head lower than the rest of your body), which greatly increases the effectiveness of each abdominal curl you do.

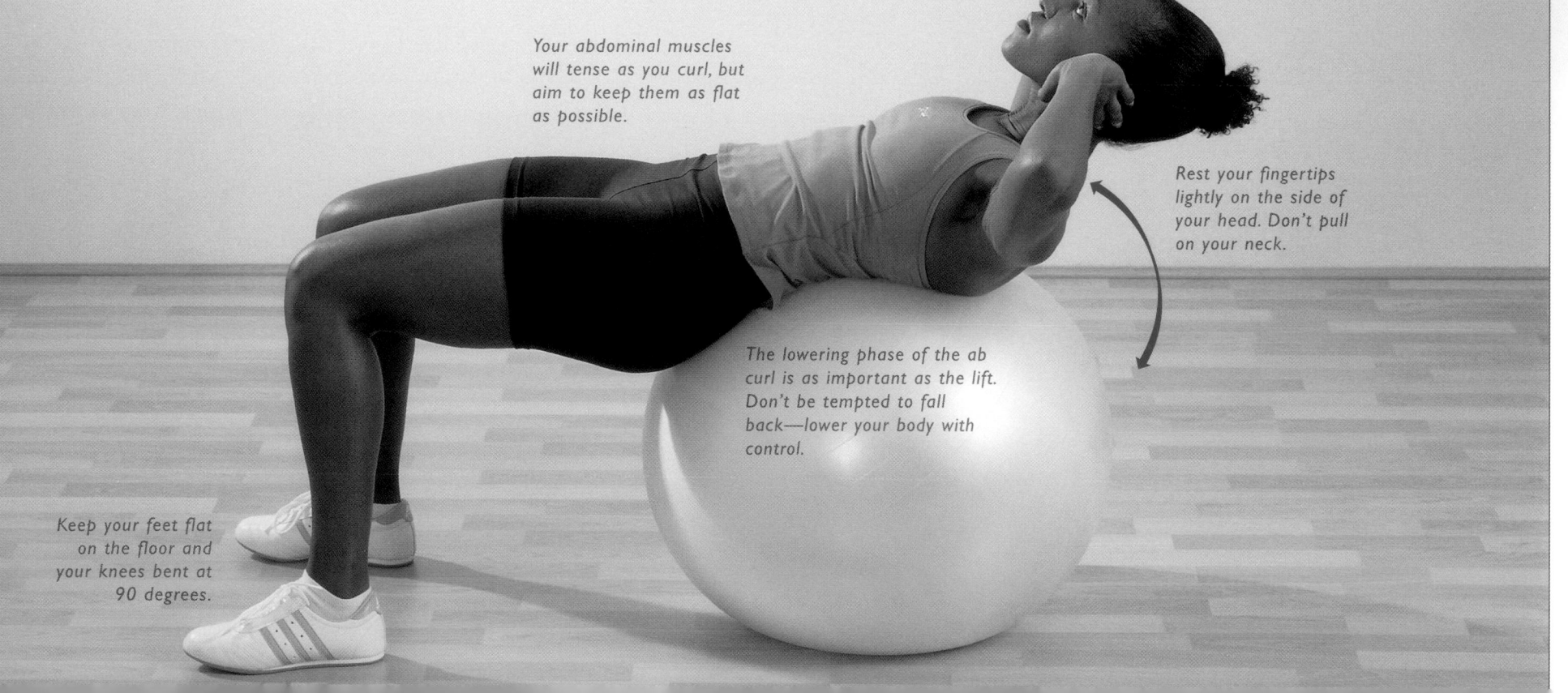

Your abdominal muscles will tense as you curl, but aim to keep them as flat as possible.

Rest your fingertips lightly on the side of your head. Don't pull on your neck.

The lowering phase of the ab curl is as important as the lift. Don't be tempted to fall back—lower your body with control.

Keep your feet flat on the floor and your knees bent at 90 degrees.

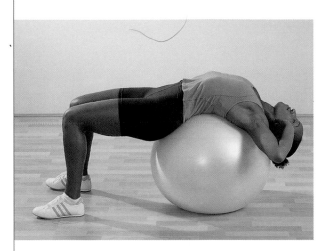

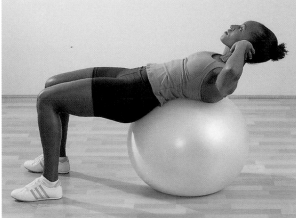

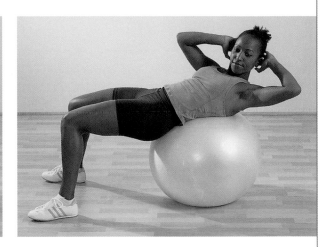

1 Sit upright on the ball. Walk your feet out in front of you and lie back until the ball is supporting your lower back. Position your feet flat on the floor, about shoulder-width apart. Place your hands on either side of your head, with your elbows out to the sides. Breathe in and drop your head and shoulders back over the ball.

2 Breathe out and slowly squeeze your abdominal muscles to lift your head and shoulders off the ball. Hold for a second, then breathe out as you lower your upper body with control. Repeat 8 times, rest for 10 seconds, then move on to step 3.

3 Return to the starting position of step 1. This time as you curl up, twist your right shoulder toward your left hip. Lead with your shoulder rather than your elbow. Hold for a second, then lower with control. Next time you curl up, twist your left shoulder toward your right hip. Alternate sides until you have completed 8 curls on each side. Rest for 10 seconds, then repeat the whole sequence.

Easy alternative

Walk your legs farther out in front of you so the ball is underneath your upper back. As you lift and lower from this position, you have less body weight to lift.

Beyond the basics

Begin with your legs and hips closer to the ball so your head is closer to the floor. This greater decline of your body means greater resistance on your abdominals.

You can also make this position more challenging by extending both of your arms behind your head. As you lift up from this position, you have to lift your arms and, therefore, more body weight.

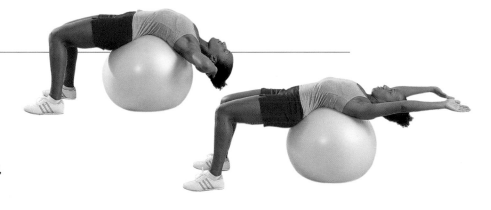

➤➤ Ab Contraction

It's good to vary the way you exercise muscle groups so you use different parts and keep your workout challenging. In contrast to the basic ab curl (see pages 40–41), this exercise requires you to start with your legs on the ball and to pull the ball in toward you as you raise your lower body. This forceful movement shows you just how powerful your abdominals can be.

There are two important aspects to this exercise: one is the contraction, which tones the muscles through movement; the other is isometric, toning your muscles by holding a position. In this case, the deep-seated transverse abdominal muscles have to work hard to keep your back flat and in line with your hips as you shoot your legs back to the start position.

Keep your back flat from your hips to your shoulders.

Roll the ball in a straight line. You'll work your stomach harder if you don't wobble from side to side.

Position your arms slightly wider than shoulder-width apart. Don't lock your elbows.

RELIEVING CRAMPS: Cramps can occur when you focus hard on a particular group of muscles. If your abdominals start to cramp, lie on your front and place your hands and forearms flat on the floor, with your elbows close to your body. Push into the floor, raise your shoulders, and arch back to stretch out your stomach.

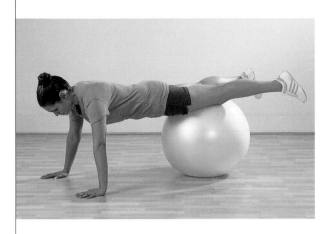

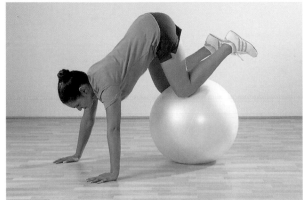

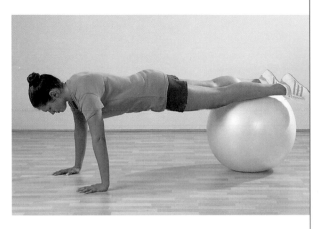

1 Kneel on the floor and place the ball in front of you. Roll your torso up onto the ball so the ball is under your thighs. Place your hands on the floor slightly wider than shoulder-width apart. Keep your abdominals tight to stabilize you and straighten your legs behind you, so your whole body is horizontal.

2 Keep your shoulders still, breathe in, and contract your abdominals to lift your buttocks in the air. The ball will roll under you until you are in a tuck position, with the tops of your knees resting on the ball. Hold momentarily and then shoot your legs out again, breathing out as you do so. Repeat 8 times, rest for 10 seconds in position, then move on to step 3.

3 Return to the start position of step 1. Walk your hands farther forward until your shins are resting on top of the ball.

Beyond the basics

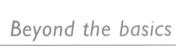

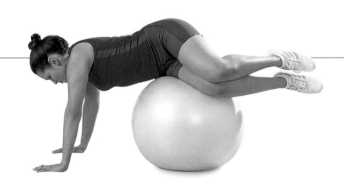

Begin in the start position of step 1. As you roll the ball in, contract the left side of your body to twist your hips 90 degrees to the left. You will end up with the sides of your thighs on the ball. Hold, then return to the start position. Next time, twist to the right. Repeat 8 times on each side.

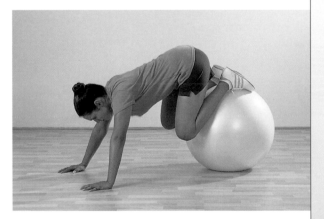

4 Contract your abdominals and roll the ball in again. This works your abdominals harder, as you have to roll the ball farther. You will end up with your ankles on top of the ball and your knees pointing toward the floor. Repeat 8 times, rest for 10 seconds, then do the whole sequence again.

≫Lower Ab Curl

When people talk about the lower abdominals, they're really referring to the lower section of the rectus abdominus, which is the large, flat sheet of muscle that runs down the center of your stomach from your lower chest to just below your belly button. As long as you keep your stomach firm, most abdominal exercises work the entire rectus abdominus. However, when you lift your legs and lower body in this lower ab curl, you feel the work most strongly in the lower part of these muscles.

This exercise can help you work toward a defined "six pack," but you'll never be able to see it unless you also get rid of any fat that hides it through fat-burning cardiovascular exercise and a balanced diet, low in saturated fat (see page 9).

Use your stomach muscles to power the lift. Don't swing your legs.

Aim to raise your hips off the floor. You may find this difficult at first, but keep practicing.

Don't press down with your hands. Use them for balance only.

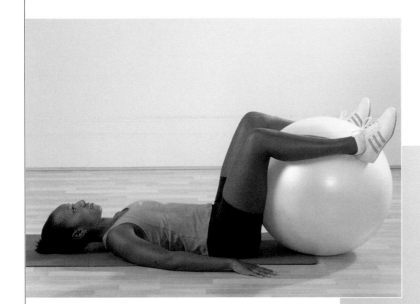

1 Lie on your back with the ball near your buttocks. Rest your calves either side of the top of the ball. Allow your thighs to fall open slightly, and grip the ball between your calves and your inner thighs. Put your arms by your sides with your palms flat on the floor.

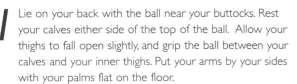

Beyond the basics

To make this exercise more challenging, move more slowly. Lift the ball for a count of three—or even four—then lower for the same count.

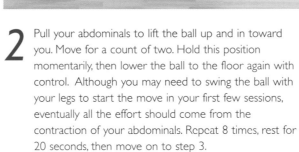

2 Pull your abdominals to lift the ball up and in toward you. Move for a count of two. Hold this position momentarily, then lower the ball to the floor again with control. Although you may need to swing the ball with your legs to start the move in your first few sessions, eventually all the effort should come from the contraction of your abdominals. Repeat 8 times, rest for 20 seconds, then move on to step 3.

3 Return to the start position. Place your hands on either side of your head, with your elbows out to the sides and your fingertips resting just behind your ears. This time, as you lift your lower body, lift your head and shoulders up to meet it. Breathe out as you crunch and inhale as you relax back down. Repeat 8 times, rest for 20 seconds, then repeat the sequence.

Side Leg-lift

Tilting your body over the ball allows you to focus on the abductor muscles at the sides of your thighs. These muscles move your leg away from your body—the motion you use when you skate or roller-blade—but they get used relatively little in daily life. Strengthening your abductor muscles can help protect your hip joint from injury and give you greater hip mobility. It's also a fabulous way to develop shapely hips and thighs.

If you perform leg raises on the floor without a ball, it can be easy to roll out of position. The beauty of this exercise lies in the curve of the ball, which naturally molds to the shape of your body—so you have a very comfortable, balanced support.

RELIEVING CRAMPS:
After a number of leg-raises, you may feel a burning sensation in your thigh. This is due to a build-up of lactic acid in the muscles and is a sign that you're not taking in enough oxygen. If this happens, stop and shake out the leg you're exercising, then breathe normally as you continue the repetitions. Perform all the steps and an equal number of repetitions on both legs.

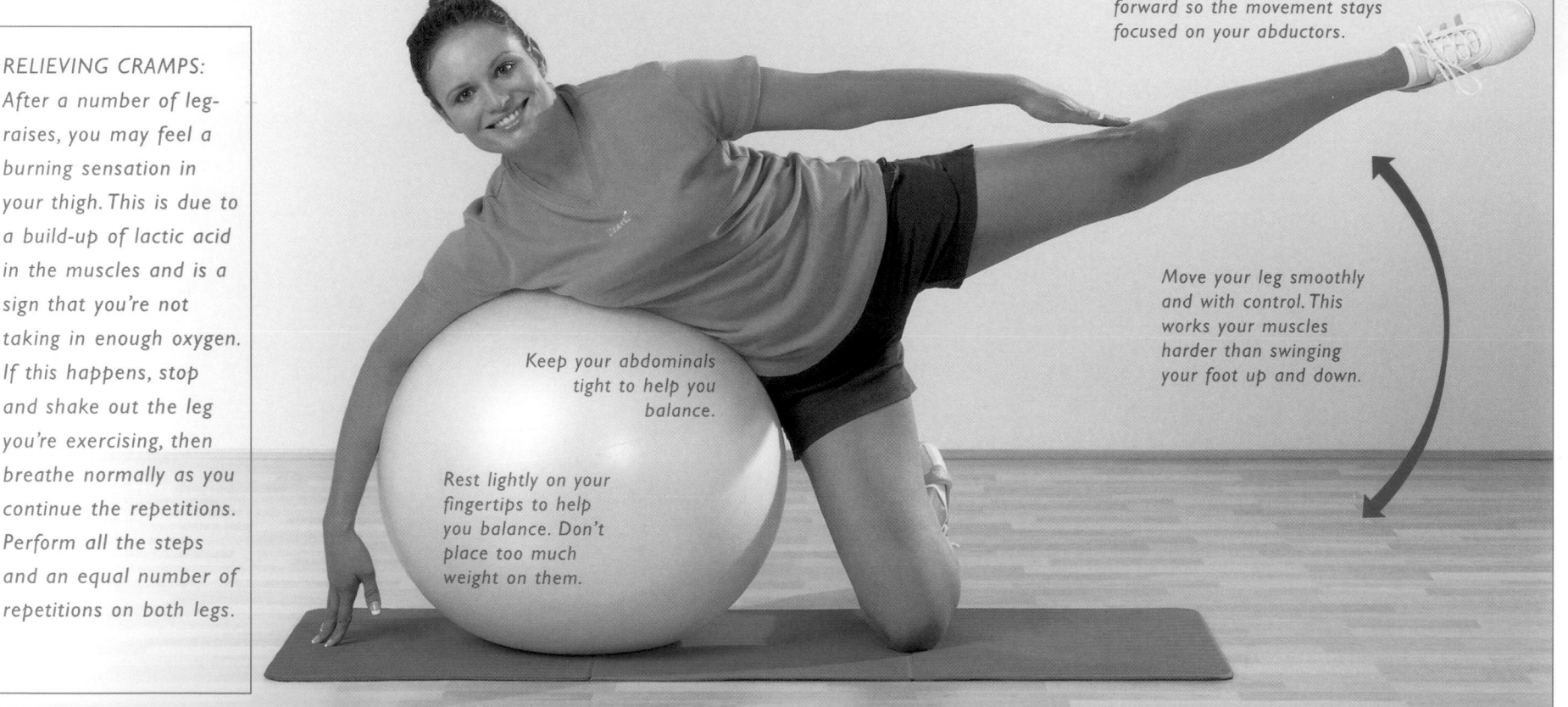

Keep your foot and knee facing forward so the movement stays focused on your abductors.

Keep your abdominals tight to help you balance.

Move your leg smoothly and with control. This works your muscles harder than swinging your foot up and down.

Rest lightly on your fingertips to help you balance. Don't place too much weight on them.

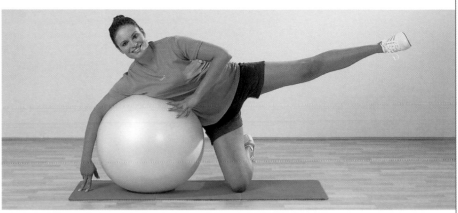

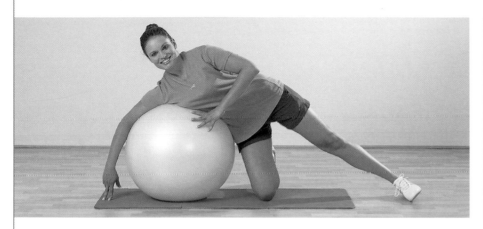

1 Kneel on the floor with the ball next to your right hip. Extend your left leg straight out to the left. Rest your left foot on the floor and flex it. Lean to the right so your weight is fully supported by the ball. Rest your right hand on the floor for balance.

2 Slowly lift your left leg straight up into the air as high as you can, but don't let your hips roll forward or back—keep both hips facing forward. Hold for a second, then lower with control. Repeat 15–20 times, rest for 30 seconds, then move on to step 3.

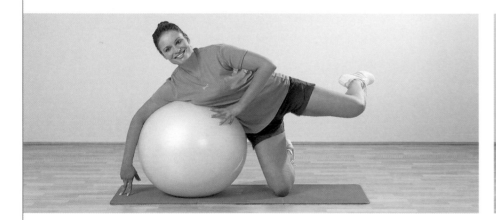

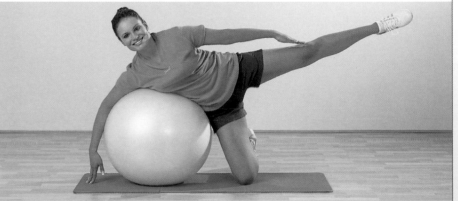

3 Return to the start position of step 1. Bend your left leg and place your left knee next to your right knee, but don't place any weight on it. Keeping your left knee bent and your hips facing forward, raise and lower your left leg to the side. Repeat 15–20 times, rest for 30 seconds, then move on to step 4.

4 Resume the start position of step 1. Extend your left arm out to the side, parallel to the floor. Lift and lower your left leg as in step 2, but touch your leg to your hand at the top of the lift so you lift to an equal height each time. Repeat 15–20 times. Do the whole sequence again on your right leg.

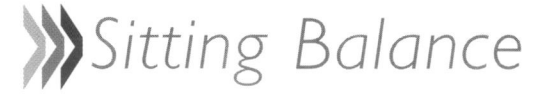

Sitting Balance

This exercise isn't just good for you—it's fun too. It's great if you want to work on your body alignment; in order to balance, you have to position each part of your body correctly on top of the others: your stomach over your hips, your ribs over your stomach, your shoulders over your ribs. This works all the small muscles around your spine, as well as the transverse abdominal muscles that keep your midsection firm. It also uses the hip-flexor muscles at the front of your hips to keep your legs raised. If you find it difficult at first, ask a partner to support you or hold on to a table or a wall. Once you've mastered this, there are many other balances you can try: ask a qualified fitness instructor to show you some more.

Look toward a fixed point on the wall to help you balance.

Keep breathing; holding your breath will not help you balance.

Change the amount of air in the ball to vary the difficulty: deflate it to make the balance easier or inflate it to make it more challenging.

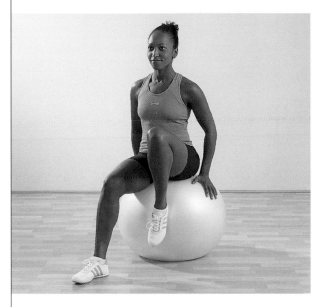

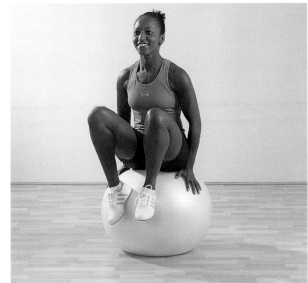

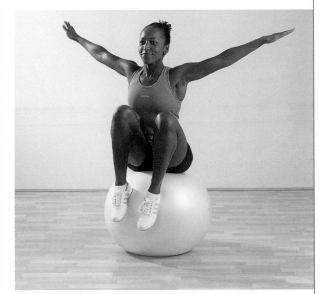

1 Sit upright on the ball and place your hands on the ball just behind your hips. Place your feet flat on the floor in front of you, about hip-width apart. Engage your abdominal muscles to support your back. Keep your right foot flexed and the knee bent at right angles, and slowly lift your left foot off the floor. Try to steady yourself and hold this position.

2 When you feel comfortable with step 1, lift your right foot off the floor as well and touch both your heels into the ball.

3 Quickly shoot your arms out to the sides to help you balance. Hold for 15 seconds or as long as possible. As you wobble back and forth, concentrate on recruiting all your abdominal muscles, particularly the lower section, to help you balance.

Easy alternative

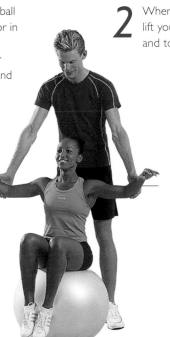

Ask a friend to stand behind you. Lift your arms out to the sides. He should hold you lightly underneath your arms. Lift one foot off the floor, then the other. As you find your balance, ask your friend to let go slowly but stay close by. If you feel unsteady, he can offer his support again.

»Butt Kick

The gluteus maximus in your buttocks is the largest muscle of your lower body. It is responsible for straightening your leg, such as when you stand up from a chair. Toning your buttocks will give you a more shapely and rounded behind, pulling it up off the backs of your legs—so this is a great exercise if you think your bottom could use a bit of a lift.

This is quite a challenging exercise: you have to lift your leg and stabilize your torso and the ball at the same time. Therefore you use not only your buttock muscles, but also your abdominals, all your leg muscles, and your feet muscles to keep the position.

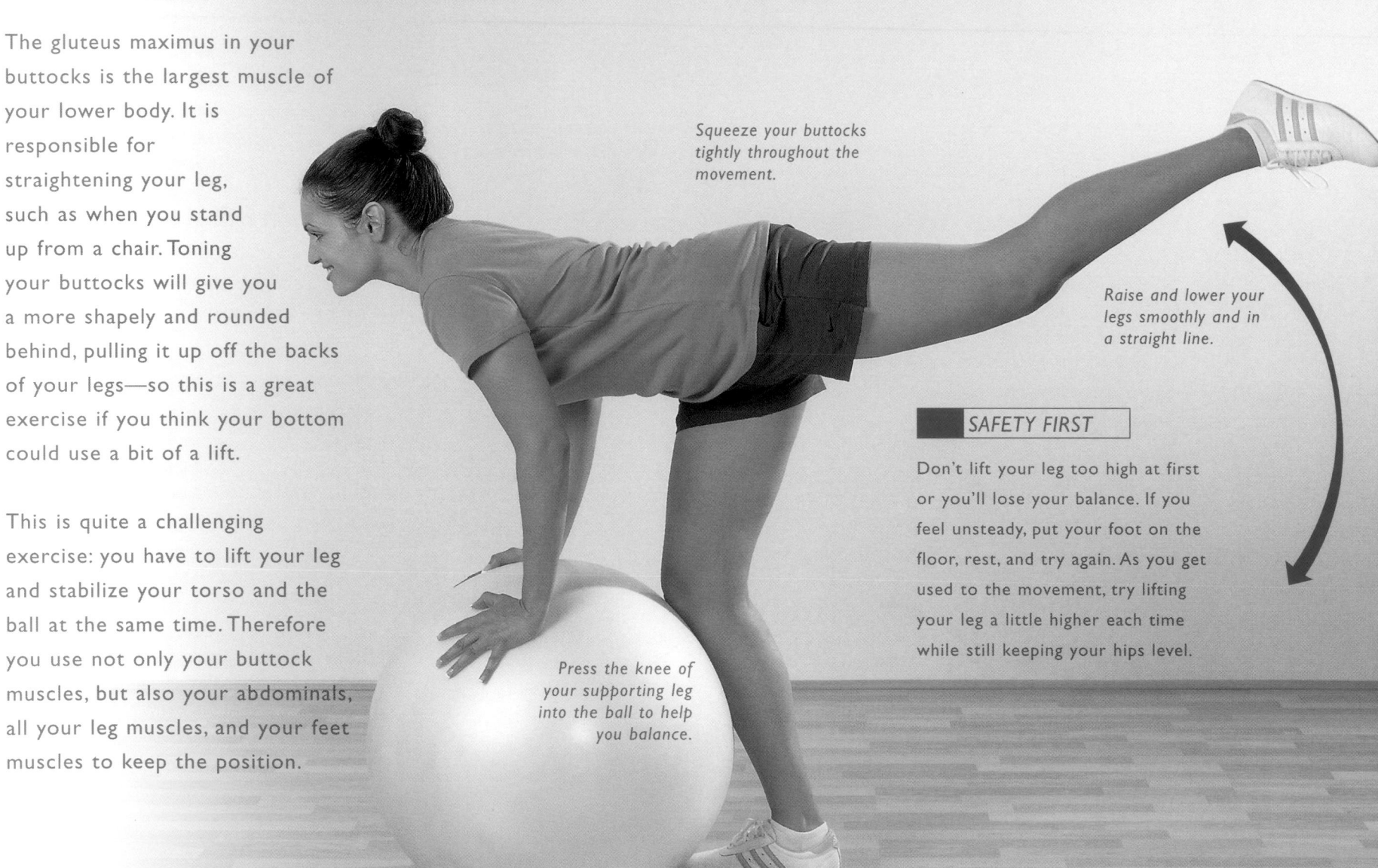

Squeeze your buttocks tightly throughout the movement.

Raise and lower your legs smoothly and in a straight line.

Press the knee of your supporting leg into the ball to help you balance.

■ SAFETY FIRST

Don't lift your leg too high at first or you'll lose your balance. If you feel unsteady, put your foot on the floor, rest, and try again. As you get used to the movement, try lifting your leg a little higher each time while still keeping your hips level.

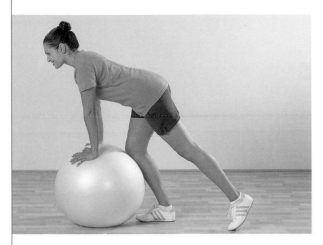

1 Stand with the ball about 6 inches in front of your feet. Pull in your abdominals, lean forward, and place both your hands on top of the ball. Keep your right heel pressed into the floor and bend your right knee so it rests on the ball. Extend your left leg behind you and rest your toes on the floor.

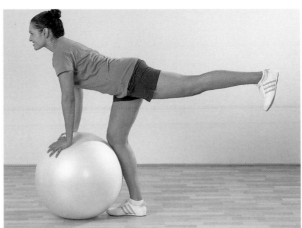

2 Keep your hips level, facing the floor and lifting your left leg up behind you for a count of three. Keep the left foot flexed, toes pointing downward throughout. Hold for a second, then lower for a count of three. Repeat 6–8 times. Rest for 20 seconds, shaking out your left leg. Move on to step 3.

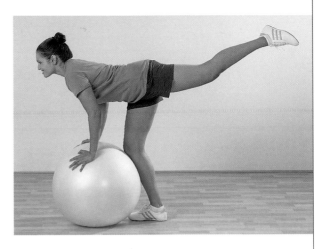

3 Bend your arms slightly. Turn your left leg out at the hip. Keep your left leg straight and lift for a count of three. Since you have opened out your hips, you should be able to lift a little higher than in step 2. Hold for a second, then lower for a count of three. Repeat 6–8 times. Rest for 20 seconds, shaking out your leg. Move on to step 4.

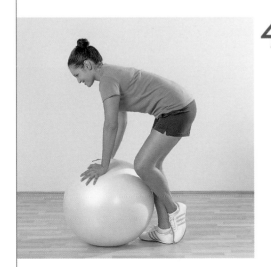

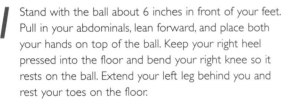

4 Keep your left hip turned out to the side. Bend your left knee and bring it close to the ball, so your left foot touches the back of your right leg.

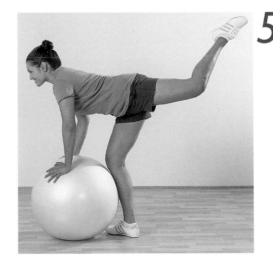

5 Lift and lower your left leg as before, but keep your leg bent as you lift. Repeat 6–8 times. Shake out your left leg, then repeat the whole sequence on your right leg.

Butt Bridge

It can be difficult to isolate and work the gluteal muscles of your behind, but squeezing and releasing your cheeks makes this a tough but effective exercise. Keeping your buttocks strong will help with any lifting and bending actions, in addition to giving you a great shape.

You may have tried similar exercises without the ball, but the instability of the ball adds another level of difficulty. Although the main force of the lift comes from your buttock muscles, your abdominal muscles have to work hard when you are in the raised position to keep your body rigid—the aim is to keep your entire body flat like a plank.

Lift up and down with control to benefit most from this exercise.

RELIEVING CRAMPS: *If you feel cramps in your buttocks while performing this exercise, stand up and shake out your legs between sets. Also clench your fists and knead your knuckles into the sides of your buttocks.*

Squeeze your buttocks throughout.

Keep your head, shoulders, and arms on the floor.

If you find it difficult to balance, press your hands into the floor the first few times you attempt this move.

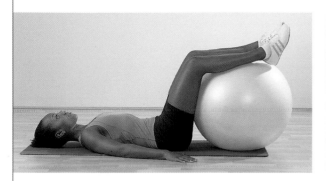

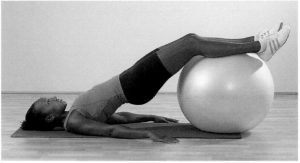

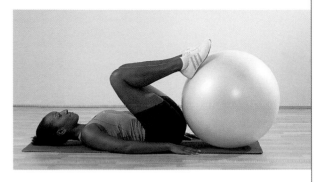

1 Lie on your back. Place the ball on the floor next to your buttocks. Rest your ankles and calves on top of the ball. Put your arms by your sides with your palms flat on the floor.

2 For a count of two, squeeze your abdominals and buttocks to lift your torso until it is in a straight line with your thighs. Hold for a second, then lower for a count of two. Repeat 8–10 times. Rest for 20 seconds.

Raise your hips again so your torso is in line with your thighs. From this raised position, squeeze your buttocks to pulse your hips upward 10 times quickly. Lower, rest for 20 seconds, and move on to step 3.

3 Return to the starting position of step 1. Bring your knees close to your chest and place your feet flat on the ball, near the top. Press your knees together.

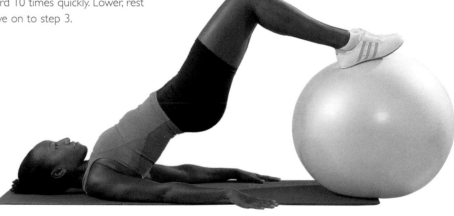

Beyond the basics

When you become more advanced, turn your hands over so your palms face upward. This will reduce your stability and mean you have to work harder to keep your balance.

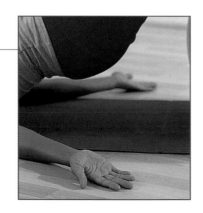

4 Lift your back and hips off the floor for a count of two. Again, aim to get your torso in line with your thighs. Hold for a second, then lower for a count of two. You should feel the work in your buttocks and abdominals, as well as your hamstrings, which help grip the ball. Repeat 8 to 10 times.

Hamstring Curl

The hamstring muscles are located at the backs of your thighs and are responsible for bending your knees. Strengthening your hamstrings can help you walk, run, or climb stairs with ease, and can lead to longer-looking legs. Because they are large muscles, developing your hamstrings can also increase your body's overall calorie-burning potential.

This exercise places resistance on the backs of your thighs when you pull the ball toward you with control. This move also tones the buttocks and recruits your abdominal muscles to stabilize you. If your hamstrings feel tight after exercise, stretch them out with the hamstring hang (see pages 78–79).

RELIEVING CRAMPS: If you feel a burning sensation in your hamstrings—particularly in the single leg lift—place both heels back on the ball and lower your buttocks to the floor. Keep your legs on the ball, and sit up slowly, using your arms for support. Straighten your legs and lean toward the ball. Rub the affected leg and hold the position until the cramps ease.

Pull the ball toward you without wobbling from side to side. The more control you have, the more you benefit.

If necessary, adjust the position of your feet on the ball between each repetition.

Push into the floor with your palms to help you balance.

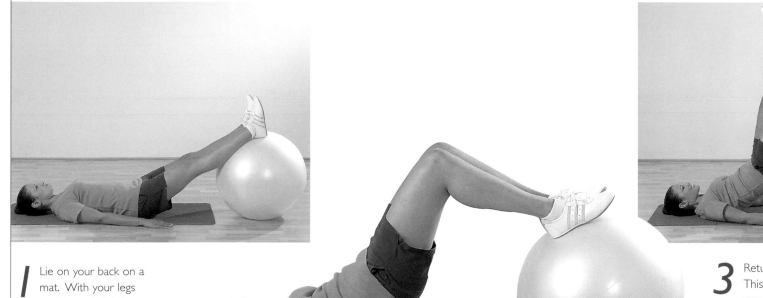

1 Lie on your back on a mat. With your legs straight and slightly apart, rest your heels and calves on top of the ball. Place your arms by your sides, palms facing downward and flat on the floor.

2 Bend your knees, lift your buttocks, and roll the ball toward you until your feet are almost flat on top of the ball. Hold for a second, then slowly straighten your legs and lower your buttocks back to the floor. Keep breathing throughout. You should feel the work at the backs of your thighs. Repeat 8 times, rest for 20 seconds, and move on to step 3.

3 Return to the start position of step 1. This time, as you pull the ball toward you, lift your left leg off the ball and stretch it straight up toward the ceiling. Hold for a second, then replace your left foot on the ball as you lower your body. Next time you roll the ball toward you, lift your right leg. Repeat 8 times on each leg. Rest for 20 seconds, then repeat the whole sequence again.

Easy alternative

Make your hands into fists and place them beneath your lower back. Draw your legs in as in step 2, but keep your lower back resting on your hands. This takes some of the work off the hamstrings.

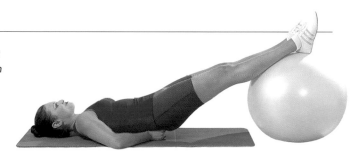

≫ Quad Toner

The front of the thigh is made up of four primary muscles, which are collectively known as the quadriceps. They work together to extend the lower leg and lift the thigh toward the chest. Some women are afraid of exercising their quads for fear of developing legs like tree trunks, but this exercise uses a high number of repetitions to gently tone and define your thighs. It also strengthens the muscles that support your knee and hip joints, so if you have suffered from pain or injury in these areas, this will help prevent future problems. If you do any sports like running or cycling, strengthening your quads can greatly improve your performance.

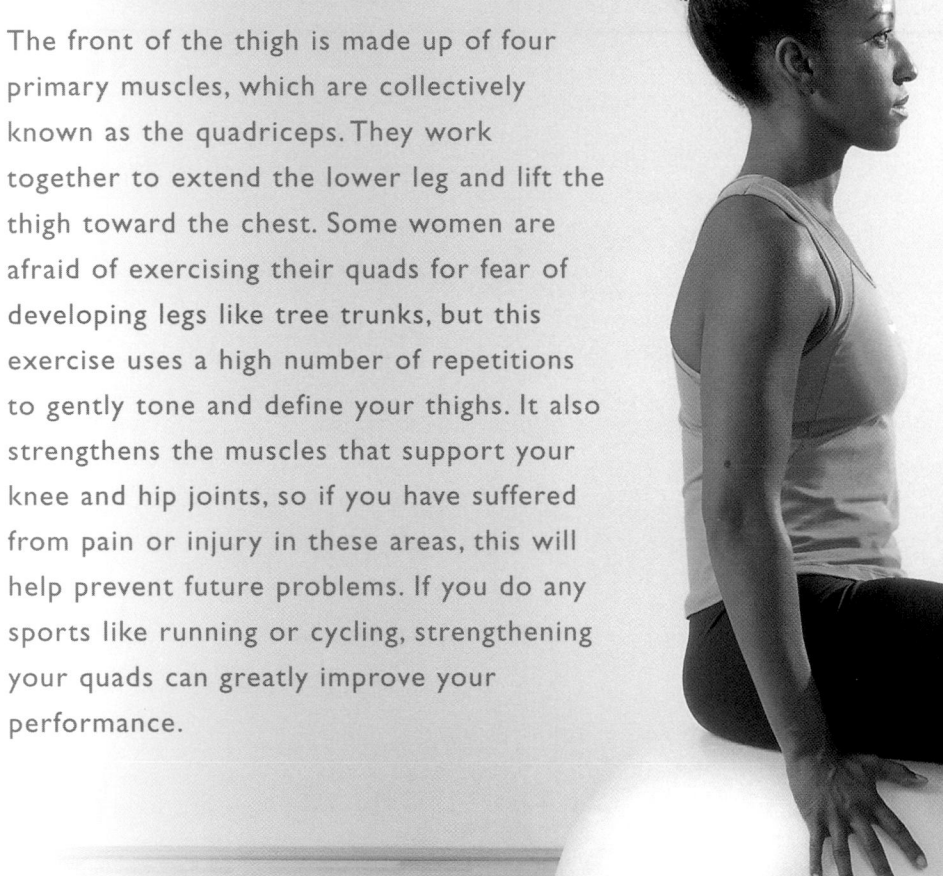

Lift up through your torso, so your pelvis is in a "neutral" position (see page 13) and your back is straight.

To target the lower quadriceps muscles, which are closer to the knees, sit farther forward on the ball.

Don't allow the ball to roll or your hips to twist as you lift your leg. To avoid this, pull up through your abdominals and your pelvic-floor muscles.

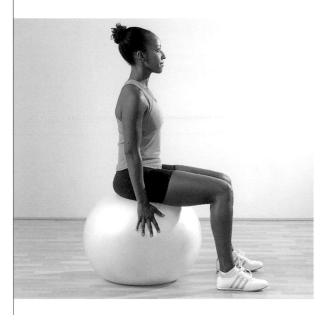

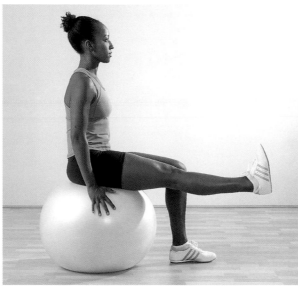

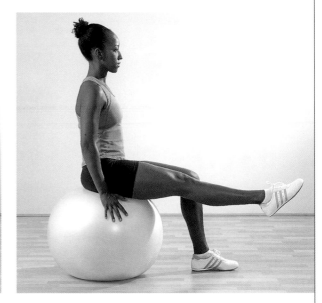

1 Sit upright on the ball with your knees bent at 90 degrees and your thighs parallel to the floor. Place your hands on the ball, either side of your thighs.

2 Extend your right leg straight out for a count of two. Hold it for a second, but don't lock your knee. Lower for a count of two. Repeat 16–20 times on your right leg and 16–20 times on your left leg. Rest for 20 seconds then move on to step 3.

3 Repeat step 2, but each time you straighten your leg, point and flex your foot once before you lower it to the floor. This works the muscles of the ankles and calves, as well as the quadriceps, which hold your leg in the raised position. Repeat 16–20 times on each leg. If you want to work your legs harder, repeat the whole sequence on both legs.

Beyond the basics

Return to the start position of step 1. Lift your right leg out straight in front of you. Turn the toes of your right foot out to the side. From this raised position rapidly lift and lower your leg a distance of 2 to 3 inches. Pulse like this 10 times. Then lower and repeat on your left leg.

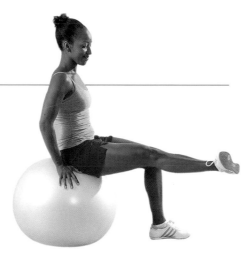

QUAD TONER

≫ Wall Squat

This exercise targets the quadricep muscles but also works the buttocks and the hamstrings. Often, when people do squats without support, they get into the wrong position, which makes the exercise ineffective and puts them at risk of injury. The ball helps you maintain good body alignment so you can focus on performing the exercise well and safely, without placing too much pressure on your joints. It is also a good way of practicing correct lifting technique: whenever you lift something off the floor—whether it's your baby, a newspaper, or a heavy box— keep your back straight and let the power of the lift come from your thighs and buttocks to prevent stress on your lower back.

SAFETY FIRST

When bending your legs, do not allow your knees to go farther forward than your toes. If this happens, return to standing and move your feet forward a few inches so you are in a better position. You should not experience any pain in your knees. If you do, leave this exercise out of your routine at first and come back to it after three weeks of doing the other exercises. Avoid the more strenuous single leg squat.

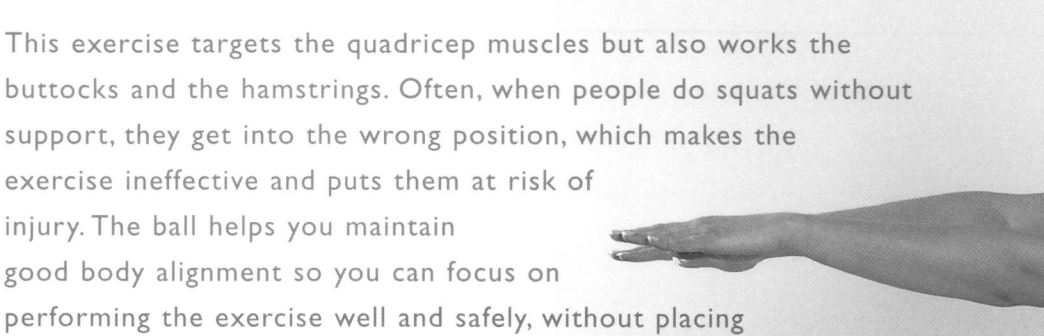

As you squat, the ball will roll up your back. Lean into it to help you balance and move smoothly.

Squat until your thighs are almost parallel with the floor. Don't go any lower.

Keep your weight in your heels rather than your toes.

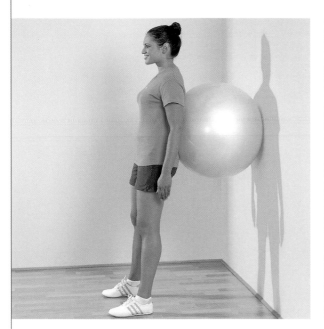

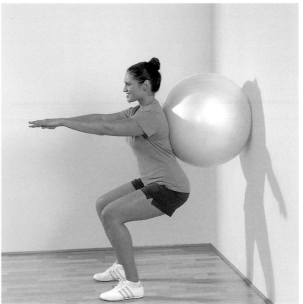

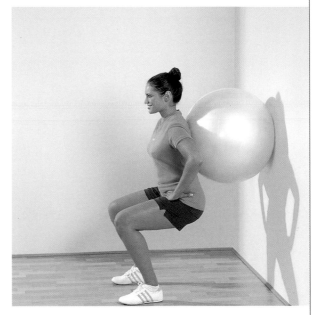

1 Find a solid wall. Place the ball between your lower back and the wall. Move your feet forward a little, until you are leaning back slightly. Place your feet about shoulder-width apart. Lean your shoulders away from the wall slightly so they are directly above your hips.

2 Pull in your abdominals. Keep your back straight and bend your knees for a count of two, until your thighs are almost parallel with the floor. At the same time, raise your arms in front of you. Hold for a second, then straighten your legs again. Repeat 10–12 times, rest for 30 seconds, then move on to step 3.

3 Return to the start position of step 1. Place your hands on your hips. This time, as you raise and lower your body, your legs will have to work harder, because you aren't using your arms to help you balance. Repeat 10–12 times.

Beyond the basics

Start in the same position. Bring your legs in slightly, until they are about hip-width apart. Rest your left leg on its toes so all your weight is on your right leg. Keep your hips level and facing forward; squat and stand for a complete set, then change legs. Your legs have to work almost twice as hard as they do in the basic position.

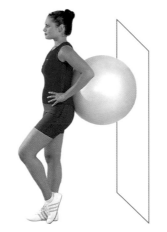

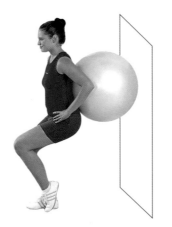

WALL SQUAT

59

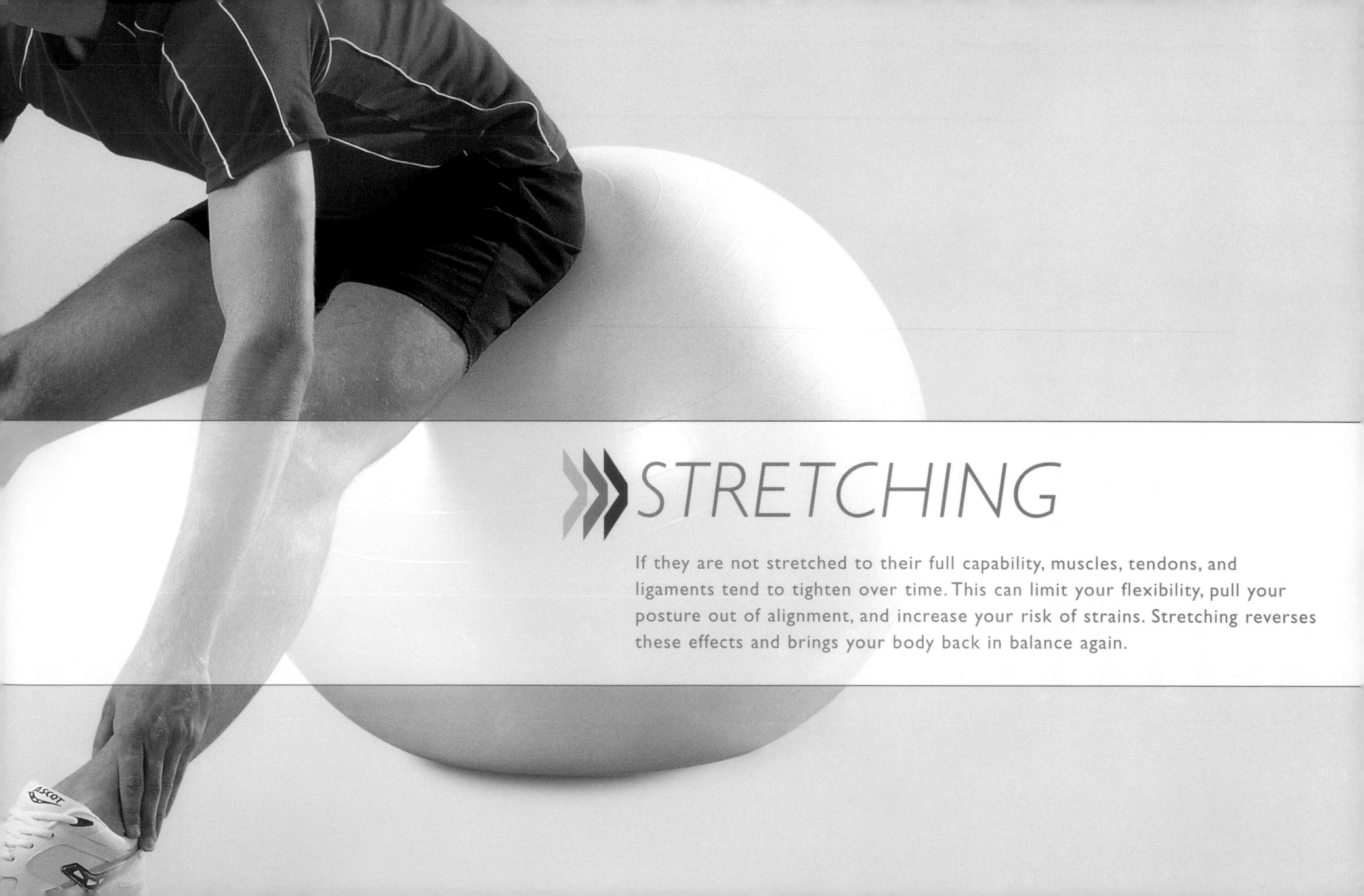

STRETCHING

If they are not stretched to their full capability, muscles, tendons, and ligaments tend to tighten over time. This can limit your flexibility, pull your posture out of alignment, and increase your risk of strains. Stretching reverses these effects and brings your body back in balance again.

Currently there is quite a debate on stretching. Some experts suggest stretching after exercise isn't necessary, as muscles relax naturally after they contract. Others even suggest stretching can be harmful if performed before warming up, possibly leading to pulled or torn muscles. While the latter is almost certainly true, the former is not. The majority of fitness professionals believe you can benefit from regular flexibility work. Just as muscles can atrophy if you don't use them, your muscles, joints, and ligaments can lose their range of motion if you don't stretch.

The older you get, the less elastic your muscles become. However, stretching can delay or slow down this process, and there is no physiological reason why a fit adult cannot keep the same basic flexibility as a younger person. So don't allow movements that were easy as a child to slip away as an

adult. Practice twisting and reaching into different shapes regularly and your mind and body will stay mentally and physically prepared for movement. You will also find stretching is a wonderful aid to relaxation, as it helps release the general tension that builds up during your normal daily activities.

The exercise ball is a great tool for stretching, since it helps you get into and maintain positions that you might not be able to achieve without it. As the ball supports you, you can gradually ease yourself into the correct posture without worrying about jarring your joints or losing your balance. Because the ball provides a large, comfortable surface on which to stretch, you will find yourself able to reach farther and relax more, so allowing you to get the most benefit out of your stretching session. Also, by rolling the ball in different directions, you can easily adjust your position and feel the stretch in exactly the place you want it.

Ways to work your program

You can use the stretching section of this book in three ways. First, you can perform some or all of the stretches after you have completed all the toning exercises. Second, you can do one toning move followed by a stretch of the same muscle, and continue alternating throughout your routine. You can also just do the stretches, to work on your mobility and as an aid to relaxation. Hold each stretch for 10 to 15 seconds; this allows a gentle stretch without the risk of injury or overstretching. If you are planning just to stretch, you must warm up first, with 15 minutes of cardiovascular exercise (see page 8).

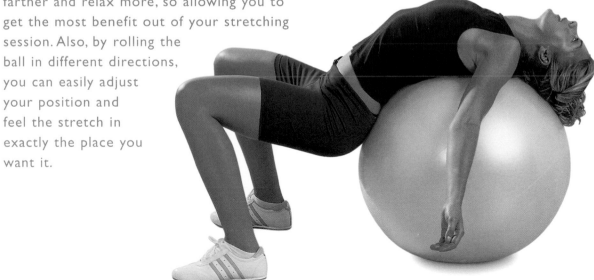

⟩⟩Arm and Chest Stretch

A sedentary lifestyle involving hours sitting at a desk can cause the muscles of your chest and rib cage to become tight. These can pull your shoulders forward and weaken your upper back, leading to the sore, knotted neck and shoulder muscles we sometimes feel at the end of a day.

Lying on the ball is a highly effective way of compensating for these effects. The size and shape of the ball allow you to get an extended stretch across the front of your torso, giving your upper-back muscles a chance to contract. Stretching your arms behind your head in step 4 will help extend the range of movement in your shoulder joints.

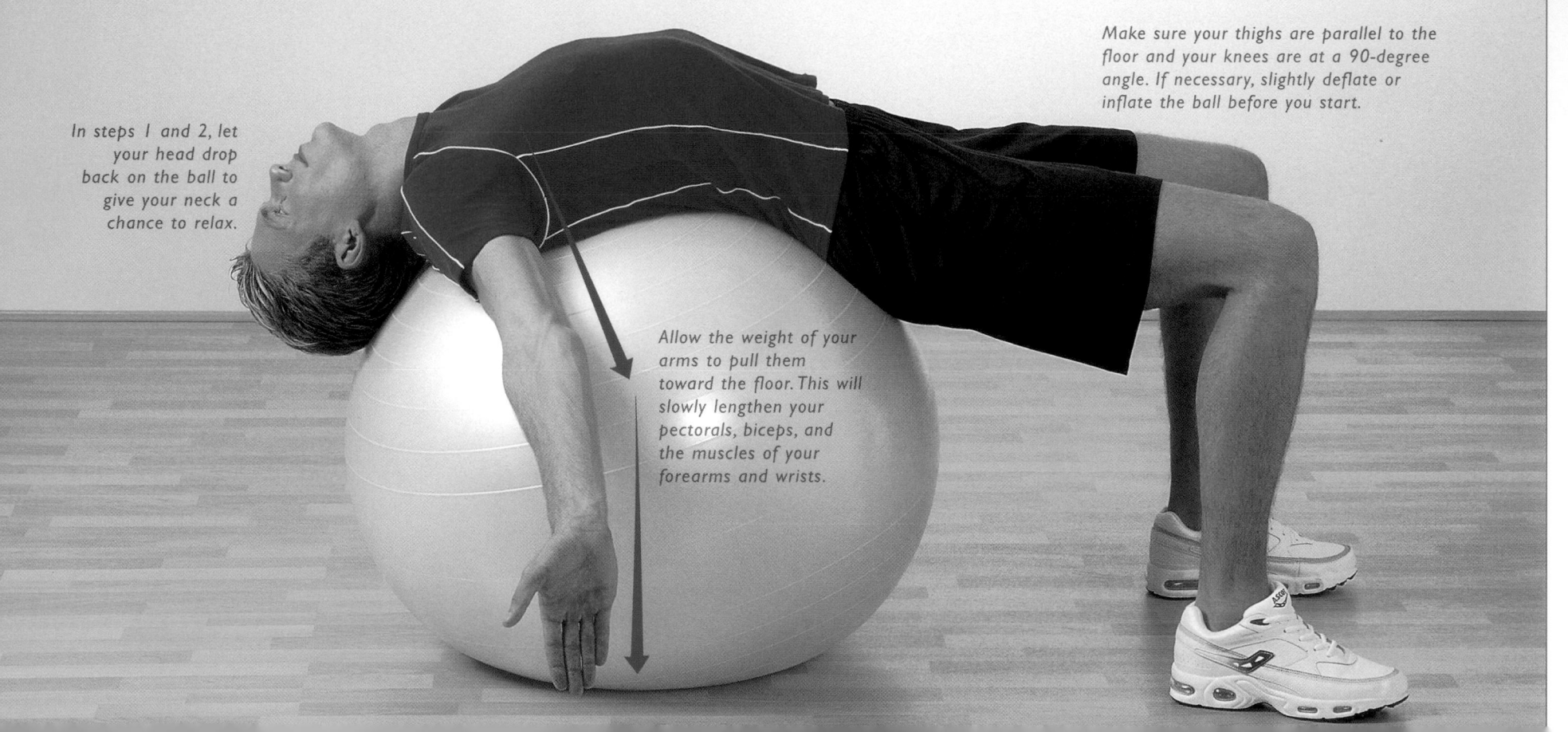

In steps 1 and 2, let your head drop back on the ball to give your neck a chance to relax.

Make sure your thighs are parallel to the floor and your knees are at a 90-degree angle. If necessary, slightly deflate or inflate the ball before you start.

Allow the weight of your arms to pull them toward the floor. This will slowly lengthen your pectorals, biceps, and the muscles of your forearms and wrists.

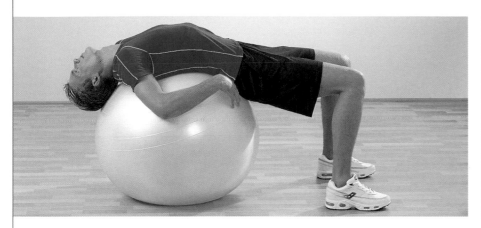

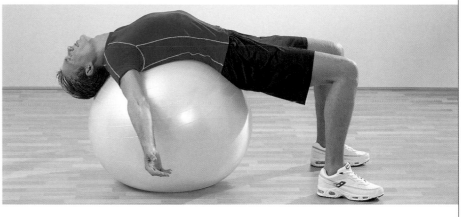

1 Sit upright on the ball with your feet flat on the floor. Walk your feet forward and lie back until the ball is supporting the whole of your back. Bend your knees, and position your feet flat on the floor about shoulder-width apart.

2 Extend both arms straight out to the sides with your palms facing upward, fingers loosely curled. Relax, and let your arms sink toward the floor. Don't allow your arms to fall too far back toward your head. Hold for 10 to 15 seconds. You should feel the stretch across your chest.

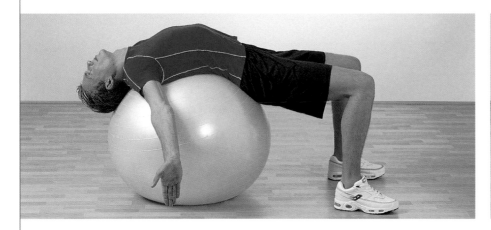

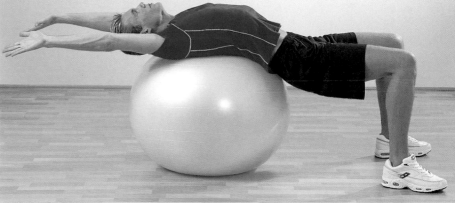

3 Flex your wrists so your palms are facing away from you and your fingertips are pointing toward the ground. Hold for 10 to 15 seconds. You should now feel the stretch in your biceps, along your forearms, and right down into your hands.

4 Stretch your arms out straight behind your head so your inner arms touch your ears. Lift your head without tensing your neck. You will feel the stretch in your shoulders. Keep breathing as you relax into this stretch. Hold for 10 to 15 seconds.

►► *Wide-arm Reach*

As we grow older we use the rotational muscles of our torsos less and less. If they are neglected for too long, many everyday movements can be inhibited, such as looking behind you when driving, getting out of the car, or even lifting luggage off an airport carousel. The wide-arm reach stretches the muscles and ligaments of the whole back, as well as the upper abdominals, helping improve flexibility in your back and neck so you can turn easily to either side.

This elongated position also stretches the muscles of your torso and chest, as well as your biceps. To get the most benefit from this position, concentrate on reaching as high and as far as you can. This will stretch your arms, too.

Continue to work the stretch at your full extension. Reach your fingertips to the ceiling as you hold.

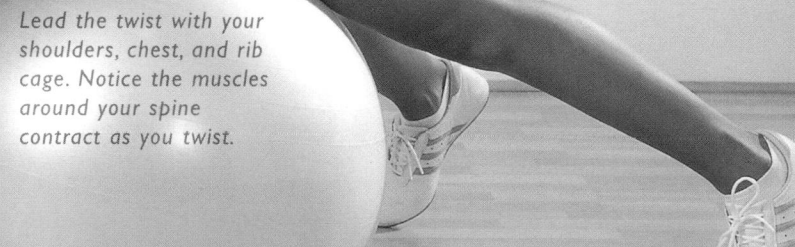

Lead the twist with your shoulders, chest, and rib cage. Notice the muscles around your spine contract as you twist.

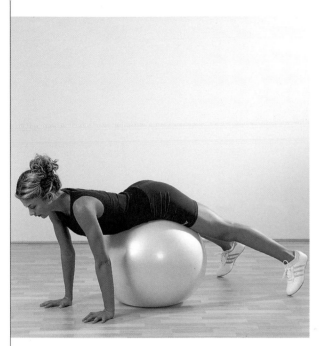

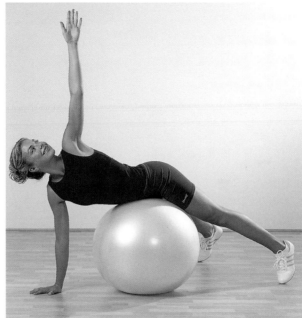

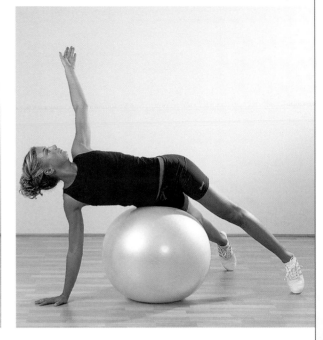

1 Kneel with the ball in front of you. Roll your torso up onto the ball so the ball is under your stomach and hips. Place your hands on the floor in front of the ball about shoulder-width apart. Spread your feet wide and rest your toes on the floor. Keep breathing, and tighten your abdominals to support your back.

2 Pull in your abdominals. Lift your left arm out to the side and continue lifting until your fingertips point toward the ceiling and your arms form a vertical line. Look toward your left hand as you move. Allow your upper body, including your left shoulder, chest, and upper abdomen, to come off the ball, but keep both hips on the ball. Hold, and keep breathing.

3 If you are flexible enough, you may be able to stretch your arm farther back. Allow your left hip to come up off the ball. Your legs will pivot on your toes and the ball will roll beneath you to accommodate a better twist. Hold, then slowly lower your left arm to place your hand on the floor again. Repeat steps 2 and 3 on your right side.

● **REST AND REPEAT**
Rest for: 20 seconds
Repeat: once on each side

Easy alternative

If you find it difficult to balance in this position at first, you can stretch your arms and chest with the arm and chest stretch (see pages 62–63). But don't give up on the wide-arm reach; try it at each session until your balance improves.

➤➤ Swiss Roll

Long periods of sitting or standing compress the joints and disks of your spine, and you need adequate bed rest each night to allow them to lengthen and recover. This back and torso stretch can aid that recovery, as it takes the pressure off your spine and relaxes the muscles alongside it—it's a great one to do at the end of the day.

The Swiss roll stretch also extends into the shoulder joints, gently pulling them through their full range of motion and encouraging natural lubrication. This is important for maintaining upper-body mobility. Position the ball exactly where your body says you need it by moving in different directions and making minute adjustments.

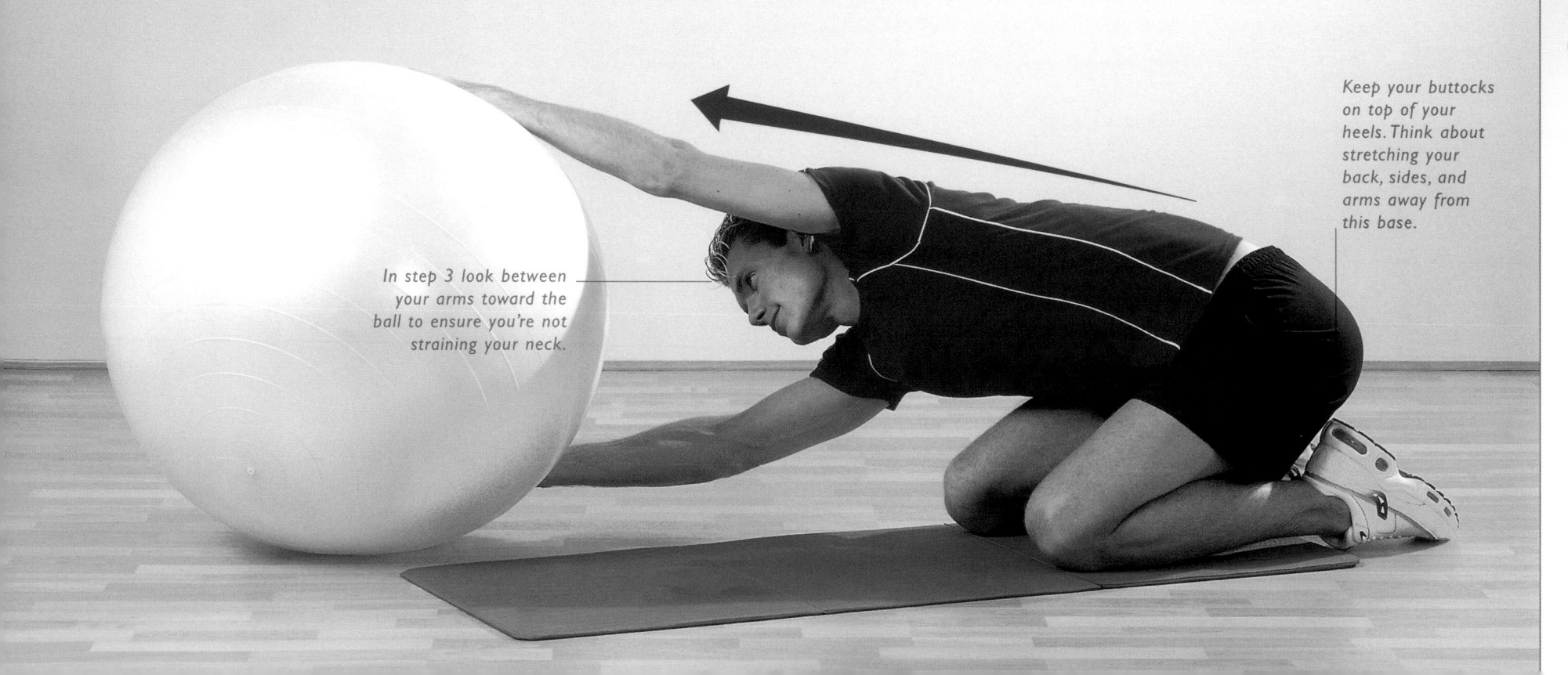

Keep your buttocks on top of your heels. Think about stretching your back, sides, and arms away from this base.

In step 3 look between your arms toward the ball to ensure you're not straining your neck.

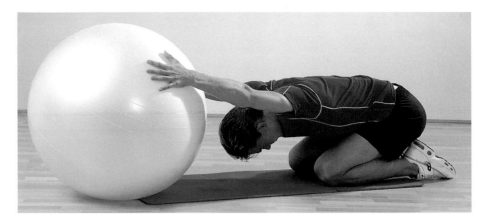

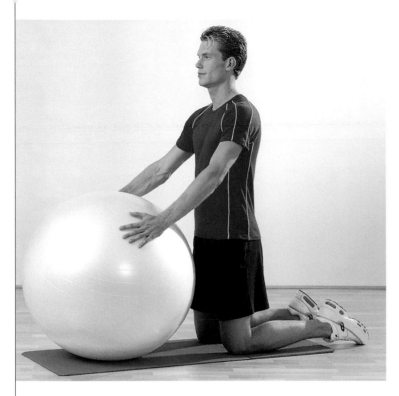

I Kneel on the mat with the ball about 6 inches to a foot in front of you. Rest your hands near the top of the ball. Engage your abdominal muscles to support your back. Pull up from the base of your spine toward the ceiling.

Beyond the basics

If you feel comfortable with step 3, slowly roll the ball from side to side without stopping. Roll to the left for a count of three, back to the middle for a count of three, then right for a count of three. Repeat ten times on each side.

2 Keep your back flat and abdominals tight as you lean forward and roll the ball away from you. Sit back on your heels. Relax your neck so your head drops a little between your arms. Hold for 10 to 20 seconds. Breathe regularly throughout. As your shoulders release, your chest may sink toward the floor. Don't allow your rib cage to jut out.

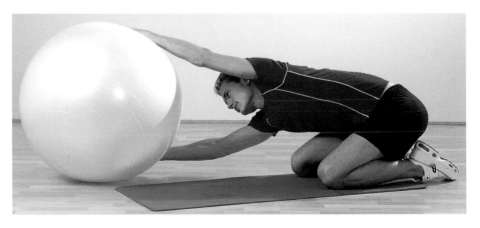

3 Keep your back flat and your arms straight. Now roll the ball to the right. Your left hand will move toward the top of the ball, while your right hand will move toward the floor. You'll feel the stretch all along your left side. Hold for 10 to 20 seconds. Breathe regularly throughout. Then roll the ball back to the middle and repeat on the other side. Stretch both sides of your body evenly.

Back Archery

Bending backward and forward is great for spinal health and mobility, because it helps the disks in your spine to regain moisture lost through everyday actions like sitting and carrying (see box, below). What's more, the ball enables you to stretch this area safely and comfortably, and it provides good support, so you can fully relax into position. The different positions below allow you to alter the emphasis of the stretch from the top to the base of your spine.

SAFETY FIRST

In each position make sure your neck is relaxed and your head is fully supported by the ball. Don't hold your head up or you could strain your neck.

SPINAL SHOCK ABSORBERS:
Between each of your vertebra, there are spongy disks, which act like shock absorbers to cushion the bones of the spine. During a normal day's activity, moisture gets squeezed out of the disks, reducing your spinal mobility. Arching your back compresses and opens the disks, helping them reabsorb lost moisture and regain their sponginess.

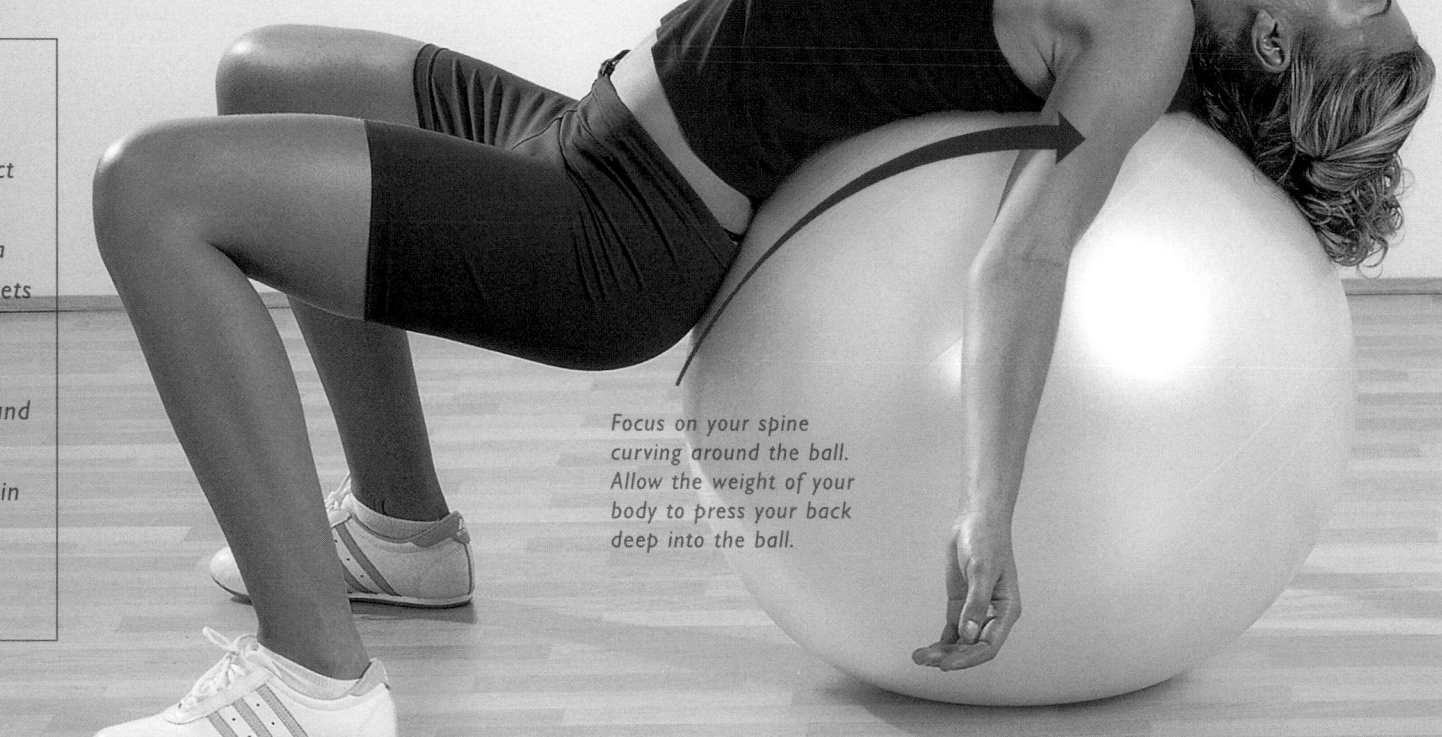

Focus on your spine curving around the ball. Allow the weight of your body to press your back deep into the ball.

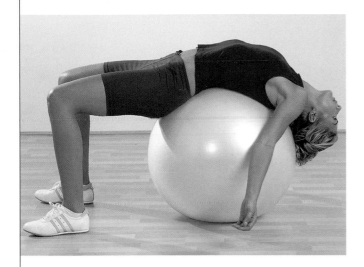

1 Sit upright on the ball. Slowly walk your feet forward and lie back until your rib cage is on top of the ball. Position your feet about shoulder-width apart. Let your head drop back. Allow your arms to fall out to the sides, palms facing upward. Your arms and hands should be relaxed and your fingers may be slightly curled. Hold for at least 20 seconds, longer if you wish. Keep breathing throughout.

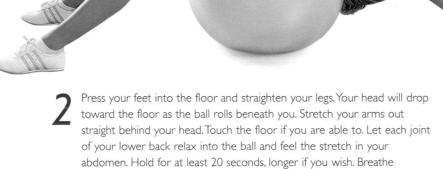

2 Press your feet into the floor and straighten your legs. Your head will drop toward the floor as the ball rolls beneath you. Stretch your arms out straight behind your head. Touch the floor if you are able to. Let each joint of your lower back relax into the ball and feel the stretch in your abdomen. Hold for at least 20 seconds, longer if you wish. Breathe regularly throughout.

3 Bend your knees. Bring your arms back to your sides. Take your weight on your legs and let your bottom sink toward the floor. The ball will roll under your upper back, stretching out this area and your chest. Hold for at least 20 seconds, longer if you wish. Breathe regularly. When you are ready, bend your knees and sit on the floor to come out of the position.

Perfect partner

The best stretches are balanced stretches. Team this with the back curver (see pages 70–71) for greater spinal mobility.

⟫ Back Curver

Too often our spines are held immobile—or worse still, forced into unnatural postures that place strain on our back muscles. This can lead to tension and pain in the back, shoulders, and neck. In the back curver you wrap your body around the ball, and use it to gradually extend your spine, giving you immediate relief from any aches and helping improve your flexibility in the long term. And, as the ball supports all your body weight, you'll find this a really comfortable position that you can relax into and enjoy for as long as you like.

Check that the ball is firm before you begin. Roll slowly from one step into the next so you stretch every part of your back.

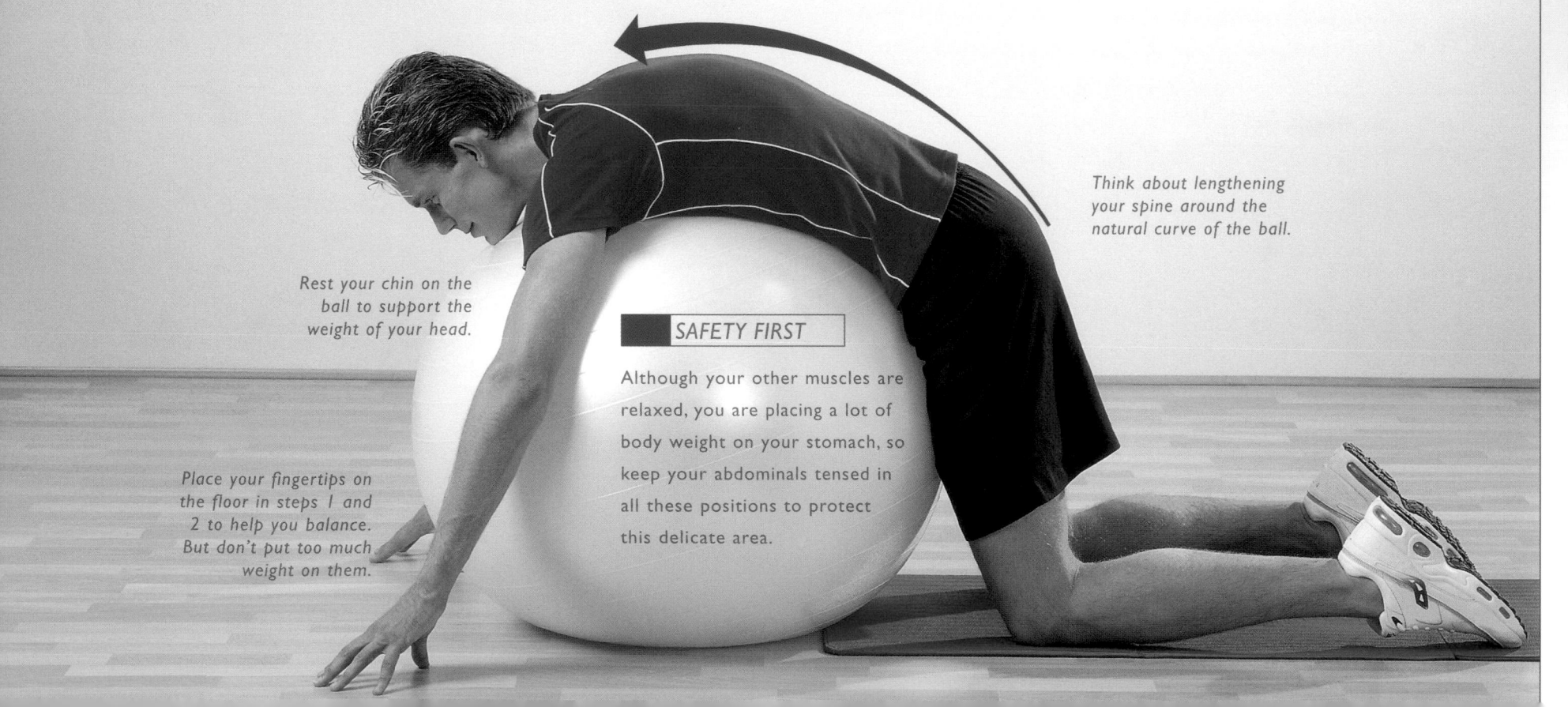

Think about lengthening your spine around the natural curve of the ball.

Rest your chin on the ball to support the weight of your head.

SAFETY FIRST

Although your other muscles are relaxed, you are placing a lot of body weight on your stomach, so keep your abdominals tensed in all these positions to protect this delicate area.

Place your fingertips on the floor in steps 1 and 2 to help you balance. But don't put too much weight on them.

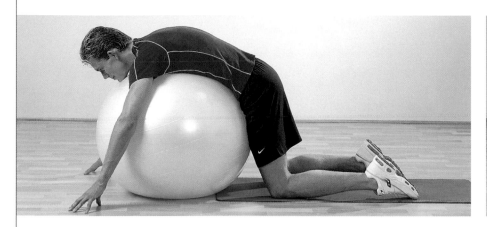

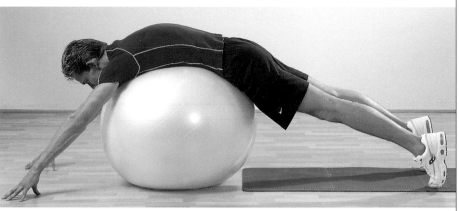

1 Kneel on the floor with the ball in front of you. Roll your torso up onto the ball until it is under your chest and stomach. Keep your knees on the floor and rest your fingers on the floor in front of the ball. Relax your arm and leg muscles so your entire weight is supported by the ball. Hold for 10 to 15 seconds. Breathe throughout.

2 Curl your toes under and rest them on the floor. Keep your toes and fingers in contact with the floor, but stretch your arms and legs out as far as you can. Hold for a count of three. Then release and sink down onto the ball.

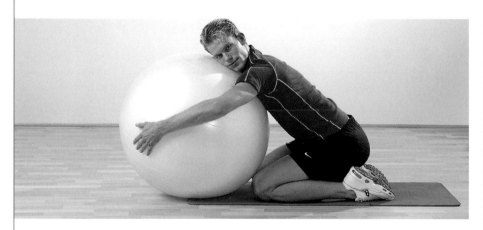

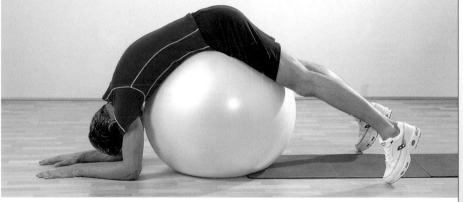

3 Roll backward. Kneel on the floor and rest on your heels. Wrap your arms around the ball as far as you can and hug it like it's a long-lost friend. Feel the stretch in your upper back. Hold for 10 to 15 seconds. Breathe throughout.

4 Curl your toes under and rest them on the floor. Push up from your toes and roll forward on the ball until the ball is under your hips. Place your hands and forearms on the floor to support you. Hold for 10 to 15 seconds. Breathe throughout. Feel the stretch in your lower back. You will also feel an increase in blood flow to your face and neck, which is great for the skin.

≫ Side Arc

People often overlook their sides in stretching routines. Poor posture or bad practices, such as carrying a heavy bag on one shoulder or reaching too far for your computer mouse, can cause one side of your back to become tight. Similarly, sports in which you tend to use one side of your body more than the other, such as golf or tennis, can cause muscular imbalances. Where one muscle is strong, its corresponding muscle may become overstretched and weak, which can cause spinal distortion and pain.

Stretching can help relieve built-up tension and restore balance. This side arc allows you to move slowly into an elongated stretch over the ball. Begin with the tighter side of your back and body, but stretch both sides of the back and body equally.

Reach from the toes of your right foot up to the fingertips of your right hand. You will feel the stretch all along the right-hand side of your body, from your thigh across your hip, to under your arm.

Keep your hips facing forward and your torso in line with your outstretched leg.

SAFETY FIRST

When you come out of this stretch, be careful and move slowly. Sudden movements can cause you to strain or tear muscle fibers.

Rest your fingers on the floor to help you balance. But don't place too much weight on them.

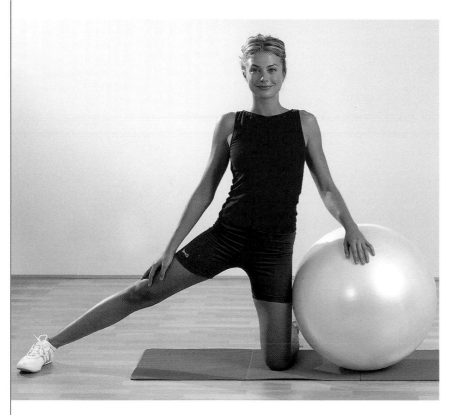

1 Kneel on the floor and place the ball next to your left hip. Place your left hand and forearm on the ball. Extend your right leg straight out to the side and rest your right foot flat on the floor, toes pointing forward. This leg will act as a counterbalance.

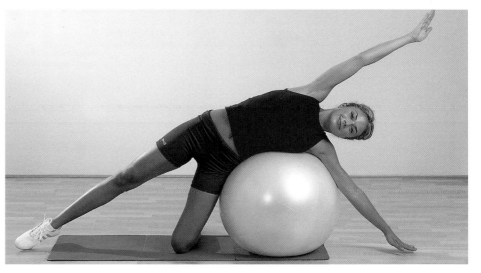

2 Tighten your abdominals. Lean your upper body to the left so you arch up and over the ball. Place your left hand on the floor. At the same time, extend your right arm over your head and reach to the left as far as you can. Hold for two counts.

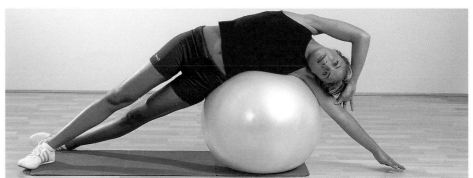

3 Relax down onto the ball. Place your left foot behind your right so all your body weight is on the ball. Rest your head on your left arm and feel your neck relax. Rest your right hand on your left arm. Hold for 10 to 15 seconds. Return to kneeling. Repeat on the other side.

● **REST AND REPEAT**
Rest for: 10 seconds
Repeat: once on each side, standing up and shaking out in between

»Lower-back Twister

This exercise is a stretching and toning move in one. The twist mobilizes your torso and the rotational muscles of your spine and stretches your upper leg. And as you come out of the stretch position, you need to use your abdominal muscles—particularly the obliques, at the sides of your stomach—to help lift your legs. You can vary the degree of stretch by how much you bend your legs: the straighter they are, the deeper the stretch will be. If you find the basic stretch easy, try the more challenging version, which stretches the outside of your upper leg.

You will feel a good stretch from your rib cage to your hips, as well as in your spine.

Keep your shoulders on the floor throughout the exercise.

SAFETY FIRST

If you have a tight or sore lower back, this stretch may cause some slight discomfort at first. Only take your legs as far over as is comfortable. Over time you can work on this stretch, taking your legs lower as your spine becomes more flexible.

Aim to touch your knee to the floor. If your muscles are tight it may take a few sessions before you can do this.

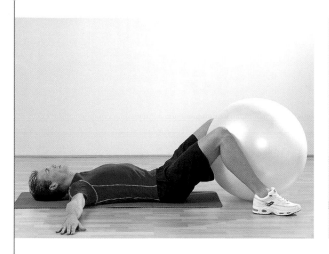

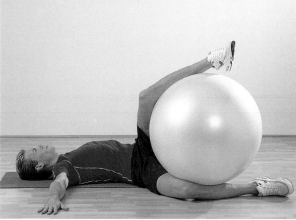

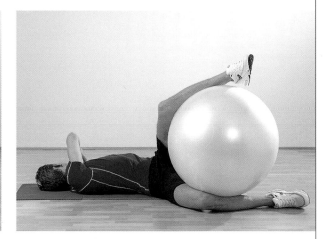

1 Lie on your back on a mat. Bend your knees and place your feet flat on the floor. Place the ball between your knees and ankles. Spread your arms out to the sides, level with your shoulders, and place your palms flat on the floor to help you balance.

2 Grip the ball with your knees and inner thighs. Inhale, lift the ball, and take your knees and the ball over to the right for a count of three, until your right knee touches the floor. Your left leg will end up on top of the ball. Move with control, and don't let the ball touch the floor.

3 Keep your shoulders on the floor and take your right arm across your body to touch your left arm. Turn your head to the left. Hold for 10 seconds. Breathe normally throughout. When ready, contract your abdominals and pelvic-floor muscles. Exhale, and return your legs to center for a count of three. Repeat on the other side.

● **REST AND REPEAT**
Rest for: 10 seconds
Repeat: once on each side

Beyond the basics

Lie on your back. Lift your legs up toward the ceiling at 90 degrees. Place the ball between your knees and your arms out to the sides, palms facing downward. Slowly take the ball and your legs over to the right. Move with control and don't let your body roll to the side or your shoulders come off the floor. If necessary, press your hands into the floor for stability. Hold, then contract your abdominal muscles to help you slowly return your legs to center. Repeat on the other side.

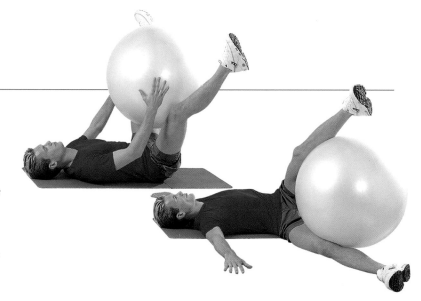

▶▶ Yoga Bridge

Curving and stretching your back keeps the muscles and ligaments flexible and lubricates the disks between your vertebrae. This move also stretches the hamstrings at the backs of your legs, preventing tightness and injury.

For this stretch you can use the ball as a prop if you can't get into the exact position, or as an aid to stretch further if you can. You need good core strength to get into position, so if you find it difficult at first, leave this move out of the first few sessions, but work on your basic ab curl (see pages 40–41). When you come back to the yoga bridge, you should find it easier.

SAFETY FIRST

Use a mat to cushion your back and spine. Speak to your doctor if you suffer from neck problems—he or she may recommend that you avoid this exercise.

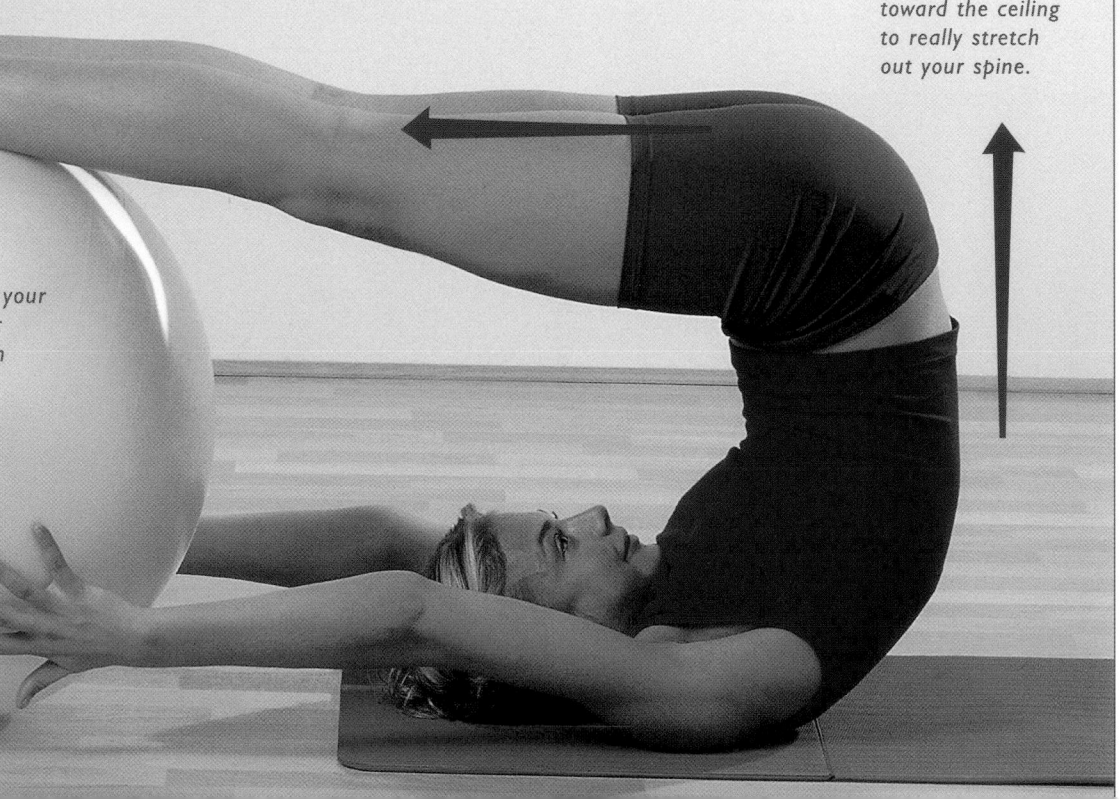

When in position, press your buttocks toward the ceiling to really stretch out your spine.

Think about pulling your feet away from your buttocks to lengthen your hamstrings.

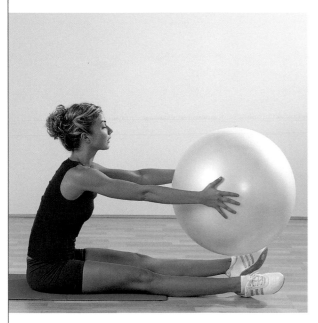
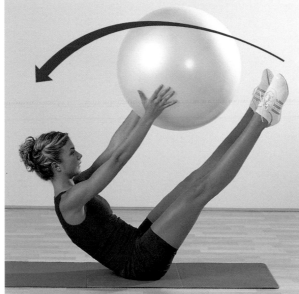
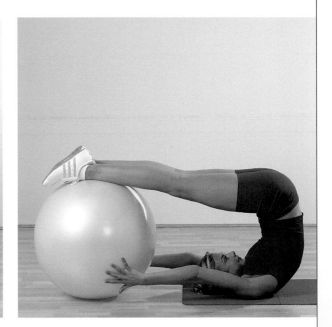

1 Sit in the middle of your mat, with your legs out straight and your feet about hip-width apart. Hold the ball out in front of you. Tighten your abdominals and lift up from your hips so your back is straight. Lean forward slightly into the ball.

2 To start the move you need to build up momentum. Rock back, then forward, swinging your legs back quickly over your head until the ball touches the floor behind your head. Keep your legs at 90 degrees to your body, and round your back as you move.

3 Finish with both legs on top of the ball and your hands on either side of it. Use the ball to help you stabilize your position. Keep your abdominal muscles tensed throughout so that your body stays at 90 degrees to your legs. Hold for 10 seconds, then slowly and with control roll back to a sitting position.

● **REST AND REPEAT**
Rest for: 15 seconds
Repeat: once more, trying to slide your legs farther down the ball

Beyond the basics

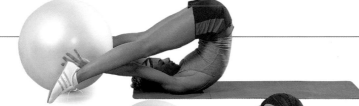

If your spine and hamstrings are flexible, you may not feel the stretch when your legs are resting on top of the ball. This time, slide your legs down the sides of the ball until your toes touch the floor. Grip the ball between your ankles. Alternatively, take your feet off the ball and stretch your legs out to the sides. Use whichever position gives you the best stretch.

Hamstring Hang

We use the hamstrings for so many activities—running, walking, stepping, and turning—that these muscles can get very tight over time. If your hamstrings tighten they can pull on your lower back and prevent you from doing ordinary things like leaning forward when sitting or reaching to the ground when standing. The hamstring hang uses gravity to increase the stretch in your hamstrings, and because you are seated, you can really lean into it.

TRY THIS TEST: Sit on the floor with your legs straight in front of you. Now try to sit upright with your back straight, without the aid of your hands. If your back stays rounded, perform the hamstring hang every day and you'll see a difference in just two weeks.

Keep your back flat and your stomach muscles pulled in to increase the stretch in your leg.

SAFETY FIRST

Some people have a tendency to hyperextend (push back) on the knee during a hamstring stretch, which can damage your knee joint. To prevent this, tighten your quadricep muscles at the front of your thigh to pull up your kneecap.

Push your ankle forward and push back with your buttocks to stretch the back of your thigh.

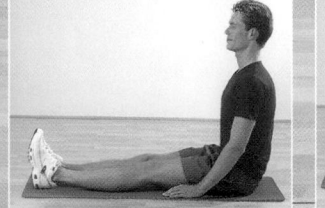
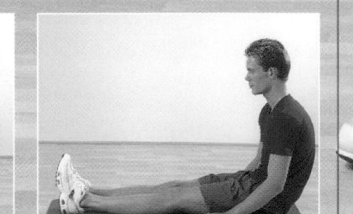

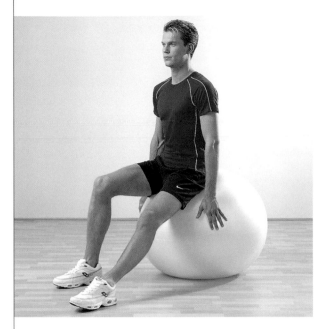

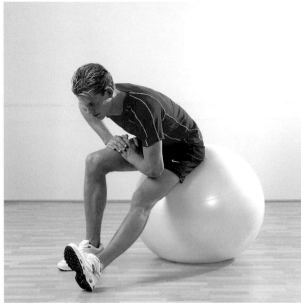

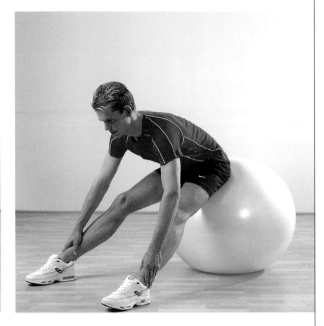

1 Sit upright with your buttocks toward the front of the ball. Position your feet about shoulder-width apart. Keep your right leg bent, with your right foot flat on the floor. Straighten your left leg and place your left foot flat on the floor in front of you.

2 Place your hands on your right thigh. Tighten your abdominals. Lean over your left leg as far possible. Allow the ball to roll under you so your right hip rises slightly. Hold for 10 to 15 seconds. Keep breathing. Return to sitting, then repeat on the right leg.

3 Straighten both legs and place your feet flat on the floor, quite wide apart. Keep your abdominals pulled in and your back straight. Lean forward as far as possible. Place your hands on your shins. Push your buttocks out behind you and let the ball roll back to deepen the stretch. Hold for 10 to 15 seconds—longer if your muscles are very tight. Slowly return to sitting.

Beyond the basics

You can increase the stretch in step 2 by placing your hands on the floor on either side of your left leg, on your left shin, or on the back of your left calf. Similarly, take the stretch further in step 3 by placing your hands on the floor between your outstretched legs.

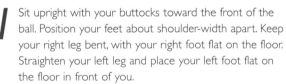

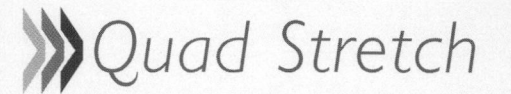
Quad Stretch

The quads get used a great deal in all workouts, and toning exercises actually shorten the muscle fibers and can reduce flexibility. Stretch your quadriceps after every session—or, if you want, between individual toning moves—to keep your thighs limber and give them a lengthened appearance.

In this position, the ball acts as a comfortable support for your leg. It also pushes your lower leg into your buttock, so increasing the stretch. If your thighs are tight, this may be slightly uncomfortable at first, so try the easy alternative until you loosen up. After a few sessions, you should become more flexible.

Don't let your knee go farther forward than your toes. If it does, place your hands back on the floor and move your supporting foot forward.

Keep your hips level and facing forward. If you twist your hips, you won't stretch your quads.

You will feel the stretch along the length of your quadriceps and in your hip flexor at the front of your hip.

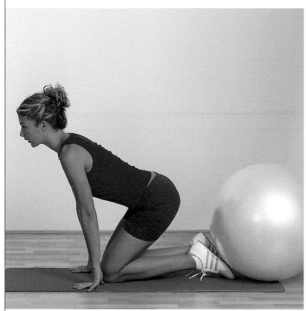

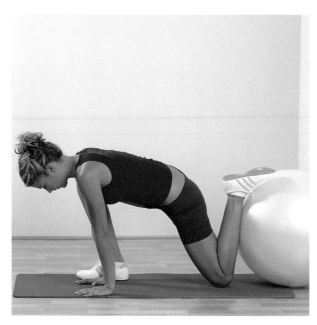

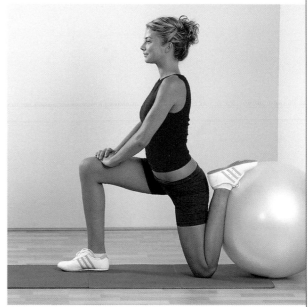

1 Position the mat about a foot from a wall. Kneel on the mat and place the ball next to the wall behind your feet. Place your hands on the floor.

2 Bring your right foot forward and rest it on the floor under your right shoulder. Take your left knee back until your shin is resting on the front of the ball. Use your hands to steady you as you move.

3 Place both hands on your right thigh. Raise your body so that you are fully upright. Pull in your abdominals and keep your back straight. Make sure your hips face forward. Hold for 20 to 30 seconds on each leg, longer if you prefer. This stretch is longer than many of the others, as you need to wait for the initial grip of these strong muscles to relax. When ready, come out of the position carefully, placing your hands on the floor to steady you. Repeat on the other leg.

Easy alternative

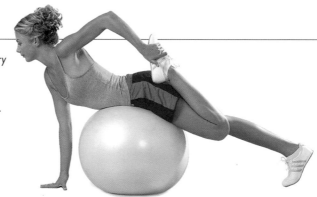

If you find that the stretch in the basic position is too much, try this alternative. Start in an all-fours position on the ball (see page 13). Straighten your legs and rest your toes on the floor. Bend your left leg and grasp your left foot with your left hand. Lift your upper body up and back to press your hips deeper into the ball. Hold, then repeat on the right leg.

QUAD STRETCH

81

▶▶Inner-thigh Thinner

This move stretches out the adductor muscles of your inner thighs. These muscles are used to pull your leg back into the body and for sitting down or standing up. Flexible inner—and outer—thigh muscles will give you better mobility when getting into and out of bed, the car, or the bath. They also enable you to sit cross-legged on the floor. The intensity of this stretch comes from the pull of gravity on your hips while your leg is suspended on the ball. It can take a while to get into the correct position, so be patient. As you work the position, you should feel your thighs release and your hips open out. Stretch both sides equally.

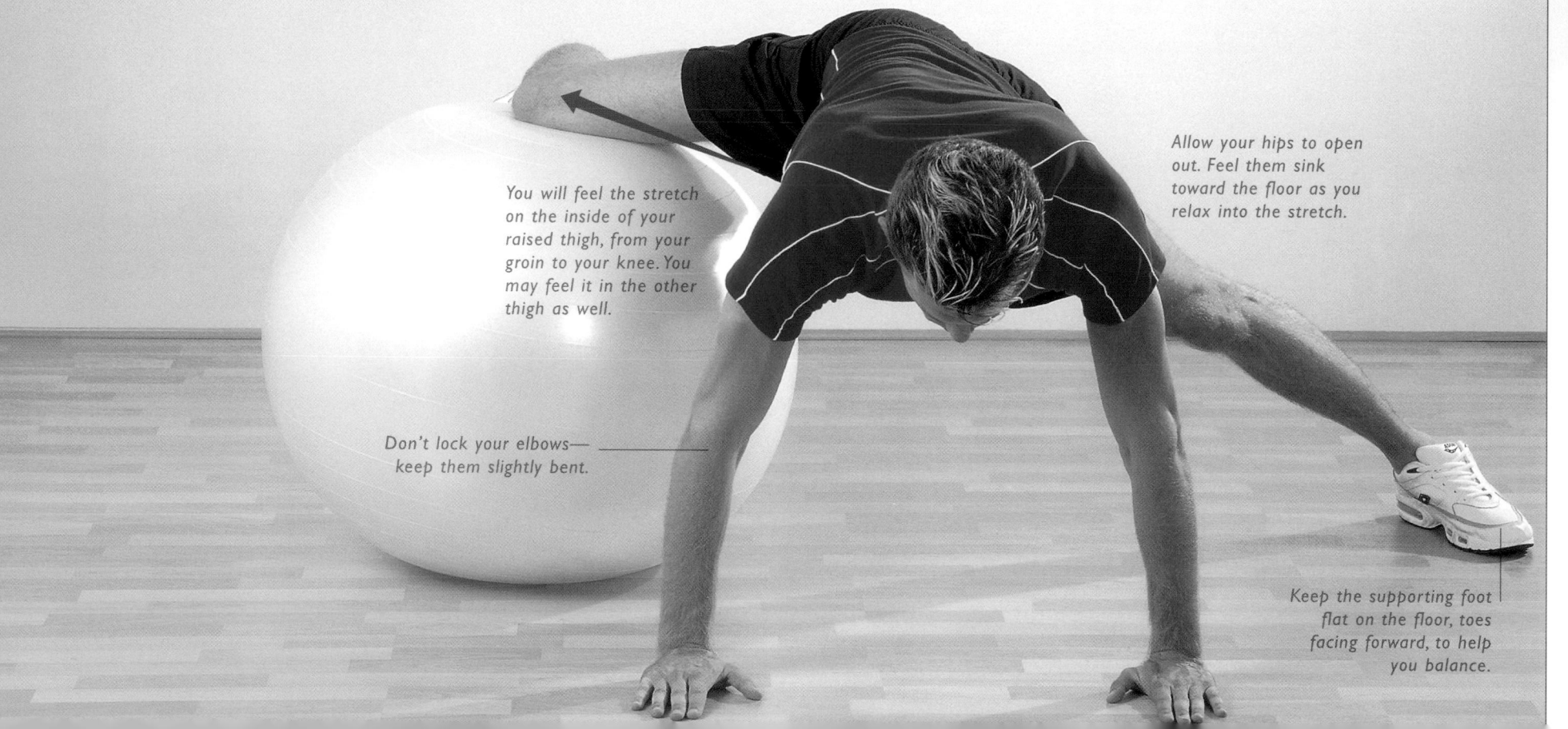

You will feel the stretch on the inside of your raised thigh, from your groin to your knee. You may feel it in the other thigh as well.

Allow your hips to open out. Feel them sink toward the floor as you relax into the stretch.

Don't lock your elbows—keep them slightly bent.

Keep the supporting foot flat on the floor, toes facing forward, to help you balance.

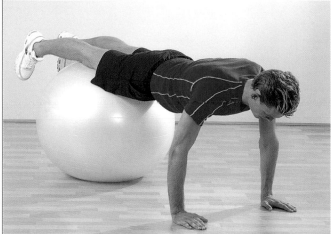

1 Kneel upright with the ball in front of your thighs and stomach. Roll your torso up and onto the ball. Place your hands on the floor in front of the ball. Walk your hands forward until your thighs are resting on the ball, as if you are preparing for push-ups (see page 35).

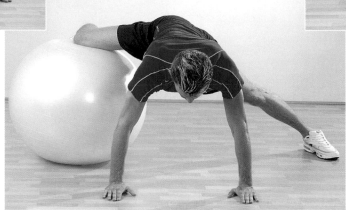

2 Bend your right leg and roll the ball underneath it so your right knee and inner thigh is on top of the ball. Extend your left leg straight out to the side and place your left foot on the floor with your left knee and toes pointing forward. Contract the quads in your left leg to protect your knee. Hold for 10 seconds.

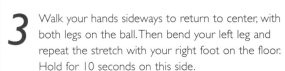

3 Walk your hands sideways to return to center, with both legs on the ball. Then bend your left leg and repeat the stretch with your right foot on the floor. Hold for 10 seconds on this side.

● **REST AND REPEAT**
Rest for: 10 seconds
Repeat: once on each side

Beyond the basics

Slide your straight leg farther out to the side until just the knee of the raised leg is resting on top of the ball. Allow your hips to sink deeper toward the floor.

≫ Splits Stretch

These positions are great for stretching a whole range of muscles: the quads at the fronts of your thighs and the hamstrings at the backs; the hip flexors at the fronts of your hips; the adductors of your inner thighs; and your buttock muscles. The twist in step 2 also improves flexibility in the rotational muscles of your lower back.

This is an easier version of the splits that gymnasts and ballerinas do on the floor. If you are very flexible you can try to do the splits on a mat on the floor without the ball: place the knee of your back leg and the foot of your front leg on the floor, and, resting your hands on the floor to help you balance, gradually lower your groin—just don't push too far and stop if you feel any pain. Repeat on the other side.

SAFETY FIRST

If you are finding it difficult to balance, place your hands on the ball to steady yourself. Adjust your feet so that your back foot isn't directly behind your front, but slightly to one side.

Lift your upper body from the base of your spine toward the ceiling. In step 2, feel the twist from your rib cage to your lower back. Pull with your hands to increase the twist.

Let the weight of your body sink slowly and your thighs lengthen gradually. Don't bounce.

These positions work both legs at the same time. Think about stretching your thighs away from each other.

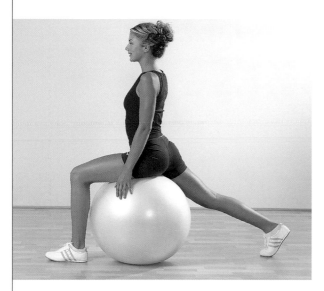

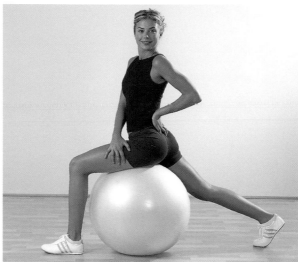

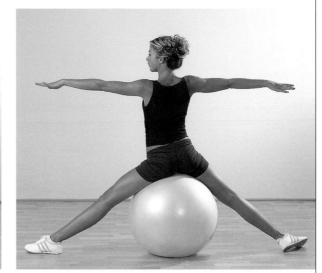

1 Stand with the ball in front of your legs. Step across it with your left leg and place your left foot on the floor with your toes pointing forward and knee bent. Lower yourself onto the ball. Place your right leg straight behind you, with your toes resting on the floor.

2 Place your right hand on the outside of your left thigh. Twist your head and your upper body to the left as far as you can without raising your hips. This will increase the stretch on the front of your right hip. Hold for 8 to 10 seconds, then return to center.

3 Now stretch your left leg out straight in front of you. Raise your arms to shoulder level to help you balance. Twist your body to your right.

4 Once your hips have rotated 90 degrees, adjust your legs so they are parallel, toes pointing forward. Allow your body to sink into the ball to increase the stretch on your inner thighs. Adjust your arms to help you balance. Hold for 8 to 10 seconds. Breathe throughout. Repeat on the other side.

Beyond the basics

To increase the stretch in step 1, place your hands behind your hips and arch your back. Don't drop your head too far back; look toward the ceiling.

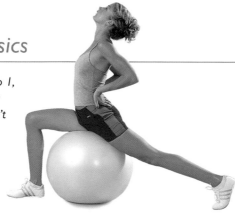

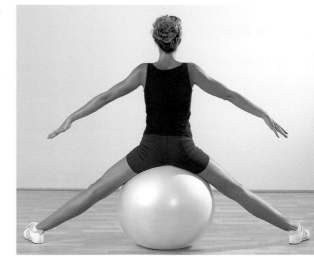

›› Calf Stretch

The calf is made up of two major muscles: the gastrocnemius and the soleus. Beneath these runs the Achilles tendon, which inserts into the heel bone. The tibialis anterior muscle runs along the front of the shin bone. If there are imbalances in your posture or if you exercise without a proper warm-up or cool-down, your calves can cramp, your Achilles tendon can become sore, or you could develop shin splints (acute pains at the front of the leg). This is why your lower legs benefit from a good stretch from time to time, and the ball provides the perfect sloping surface on which to do this. These two positions are a great complement to each other, stretching both the fronts and backs of the lower legs.

Keep the knee of your supporting leg slightly bent.

Feel the stretch along the length of your calf, from the back of your knee and down into your Achilles tendon.

Push your heel into the ball to increase the stretch.

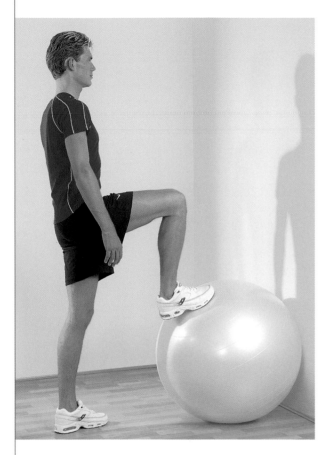

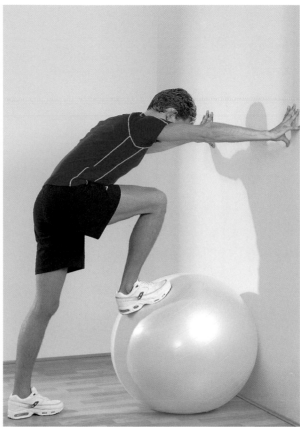

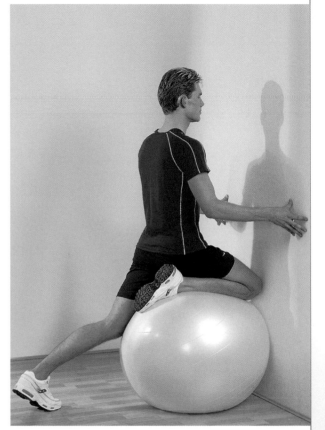

1 Place the ball against a wall. Stand facing the ball, about 2 feet away, with your feet hip-width apart and your toes pointing forward. Bend your knees slightly. Lift your right leg and place your right foot high up on the ball—but not on top of it.

2 Tighten your abdominals, keep your back flat, and lean over your right leg. This will increase the bend in your knee. Rest your hands on the wall to help you balance. Hold for 10 to 15 seconds. Replace your right leg on the floor. Repeat on the left leg.

3 Return to the start position. Bend your right knee and rest your right shin on top of the ball. Place your hands on the wall. Check that your ankle and the top of your foot are on the ball. Keep your left foot on the floor, but place your weight on your right leg. Feel the stretch along your right shin and ankle. Hold for 10 to 15 seconds. Return to standing. Repeat with the left leg.

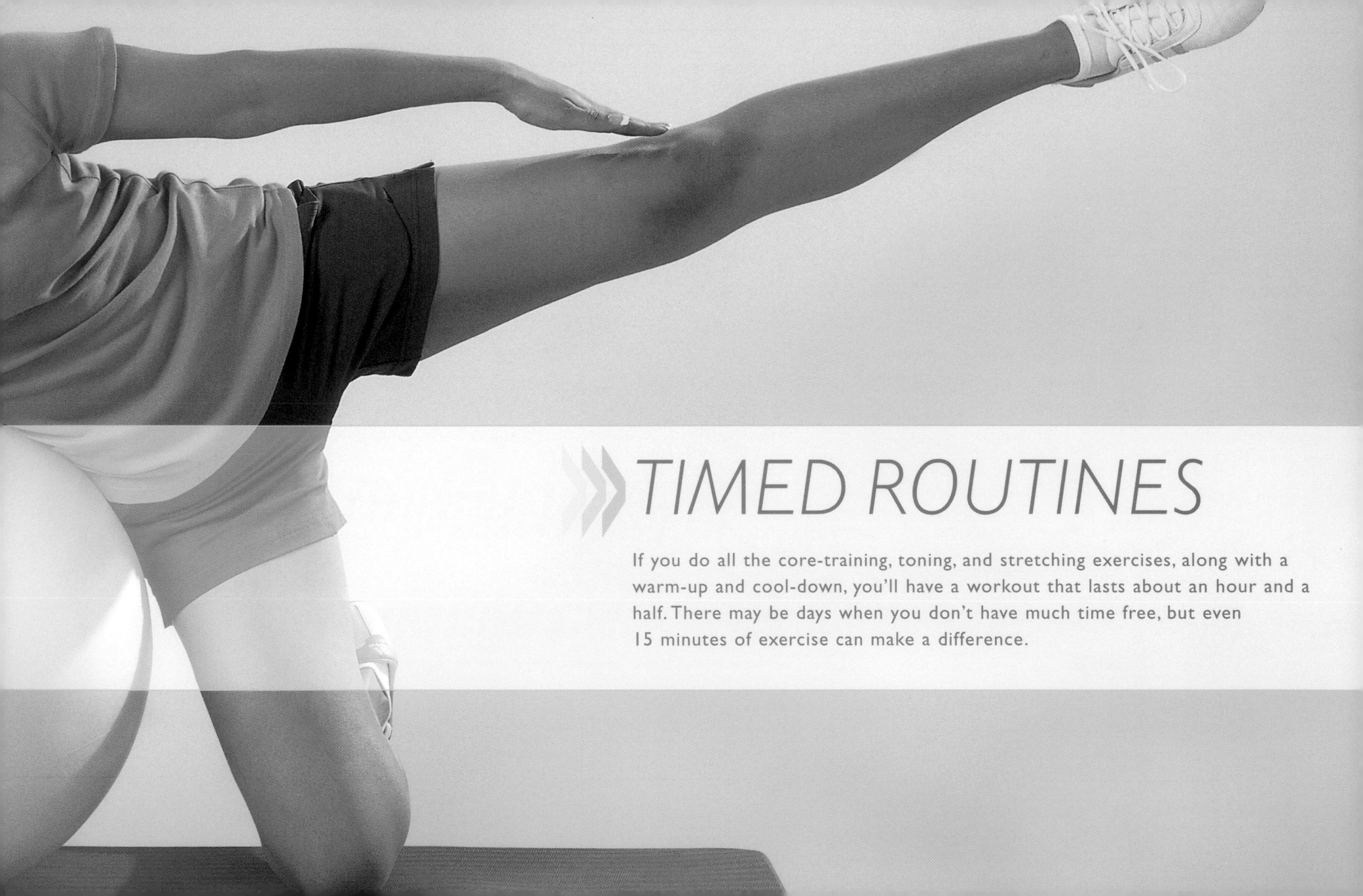

»TIMED ROUTINES

If you do all the core-training, toning, and stretching exercises, along with a warm-up and cool-down, you'll have a workout that lasts about an hour and a half. There may be days when you don't have much time free, but even 15 minutes of exercise can make a difference.

If you are trying to tone up quickly then you should aim to exercise every other day. A 15-, 30-, or 45-minute workout every two or three days will give you much better results than if you exercise for two hours only once a week. If you are feeling tired or unmotivated on a particular day, resist the urge to skip your workout. Try saying to yourself, "I will do just two toning exercises and two stretches." The minute you get moving, you'll probably feel energized, and will find it easy to add in a few more moves.

Design your own workout

If you don't want to follow one of the suggested routines, you can design your own workout, but try to include exercises from each part of the book. You need to begin with a good warm-up each time you exercise on the ball. This will get your blood

flowing and will literally warm your muscles so you can tone and stretch more easily and reduce your risk of strain or injury. Your warm-up can consist of either the routine on pages 14–17 or of 5 to 10 minutes of gentle cardiovascular exercise, such as cycling, running, or brisk walking. If you regularly do a cardiovascular workout anyway, you can save time by doing your ball workout immediately afterward.

Follow the warm-up with the core-training moves. These will remind you each time of the importance of posture and correct positioning, so that you don't slip into bad habits as the weeks go by.

Next, work through the toning moves. You can perform one set of each toning exercise in turn until you have finished them all. Then, if you like, start from the top again and repeat the sequence a second, or even a third, time. The second option is to do one set of repetitions for each exercise, take the recommended break, then do another set of the same moves before moving on to the next.

After the toning session, the stretches are a great way to relax your body and improve your flexibility. They will also help prevent injury and muscle soreness. If you don't follow the routines suggested on the following pages, make sure you stretch out the same muscles you've been toning.

Finally, perform the cool-down moves (see pages 18–19). These will relax and invigorate you for the rest of the day.

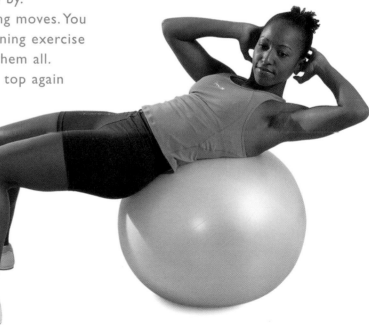

The 15-minute Routine

If you haven't got time for a whole hour of exercise or don't feel you can exercise for that long, even 15 minutes on the ball can be of benefit—it is important if you want to develop muscle tone and flexibility that you do some sort of activity regularly. A short version of the workout will also help you stay in touch with all the moves so you don't forget good technique. When you have more time, go back to a fuller version of the routine.

Follow the recommendations for repetitions and sets given with each exercise. Don't worry if you can't do it in 15 minutes at first; you should speed up as you get used to the moves. If you still can't manage all the exercises in the time, do fewer repetitions or sets, but make sure you tone and stretch each side of your body evenly.

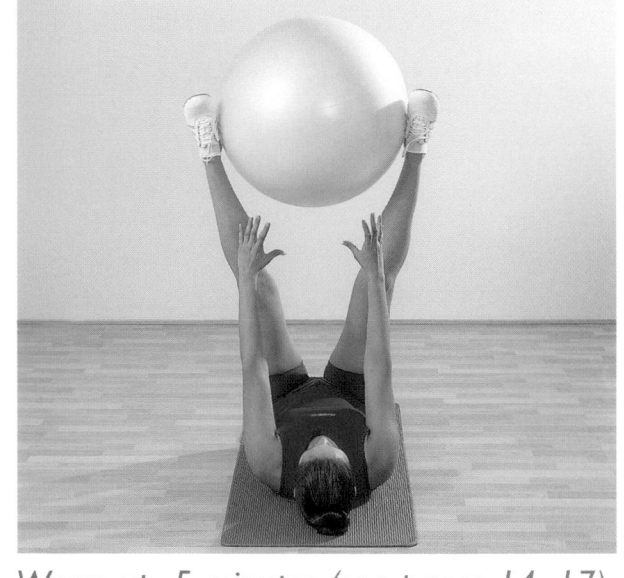

Warm up, 5 minutes (see pages 14–17)

The plank (see pages 30–31)
Hold for 10 seconds ⇒ repeat twice more

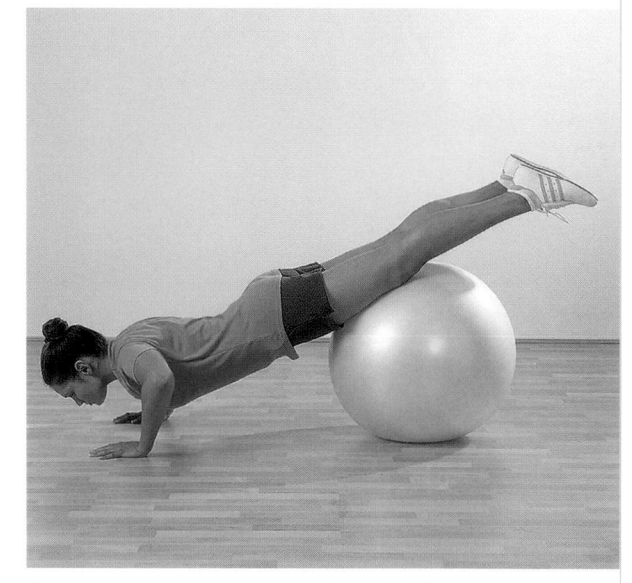

Push-up (see pages 34–35)
10-12 then add't'l 10-12 w/ arms
just wider than shoulder width

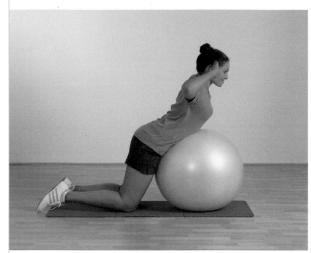

Back toner *(see pages 38–39)*

Lift for 2, hold for 2 ⇒ 16 reps
Repeat w/ arms out to sides balancing on ball

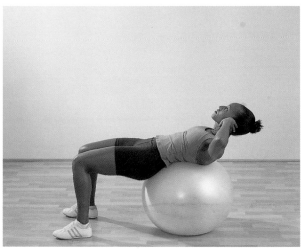

Basic ab curl *(see pages 40–41)*

8 reps, 8 alternating curls ⇒ repeat entire sequence

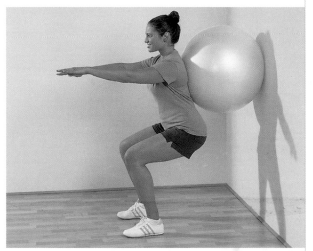

Wall squat *(see pages 58–59)*

10-12 reps repeat another 10-12 reps w/ hands on hips

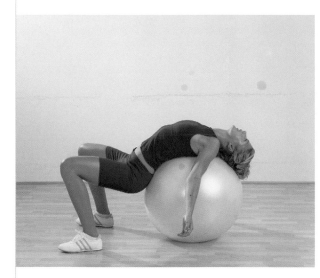

Back archery *(see pages 68–69)*

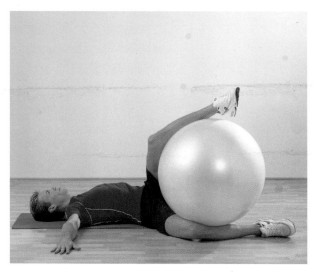

Lower-back twister *(see pages 74–75)*

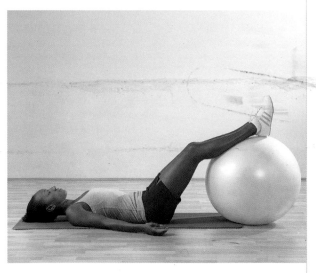

Cool-down: leg elevation *(see page 19)*

»»» *The 30-minute Routine*

If you complete a 30-minute routine every other day, you will soon notice the benefits. However, you should try to fit in a longer routine at least once a week. Follow the recommendations for repetitions and rests given with each exercise. Don't worry if you can't do it in 30 minutes at first—you should speed up as you get used to the moves.

If you're doing lots of 30-minute routines, try to swap some of the moves suggested here for exercises that work different parts of your body. Although you may want to concentrate on getting a flat stomach, you'll get better health and weight-loss benefits from all-over muscle strengthening (see page 33) as you keep challenging your body in different ways.

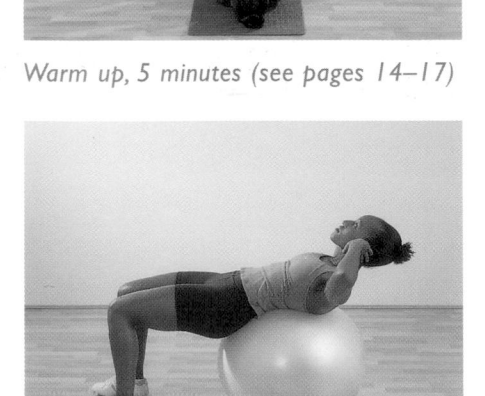

Warm up, 5 minutes (see pages 14–17)

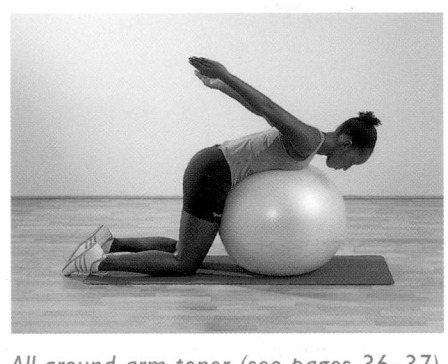

Push-up (see pages 34–35)

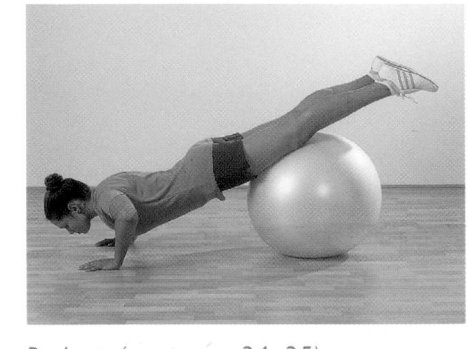

All-around arm toner (see pages 36–37)

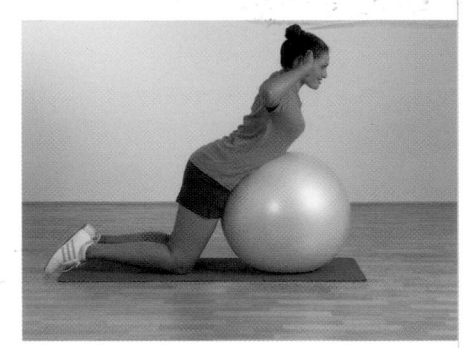

Back toner (see pages 38–39)

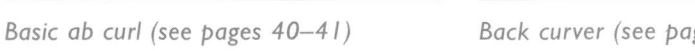

Basic ab curl (see pages 40–41)

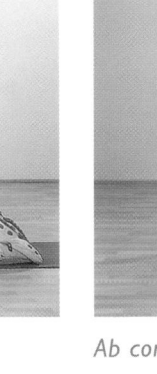

Back curver (see pages 70–71)

Ab contraction (see pages 42–43)

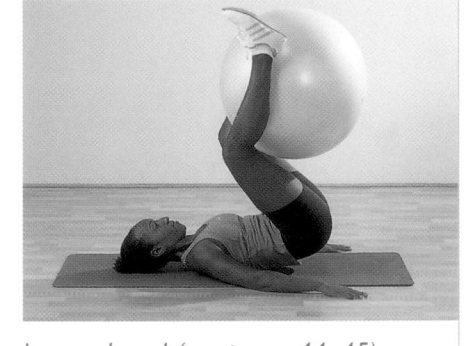

Lower ab curl (see pages 44–45)

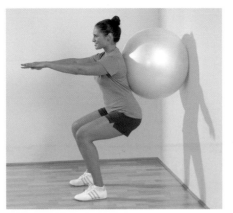

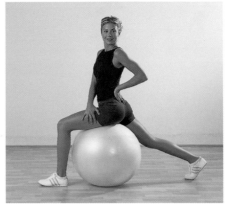

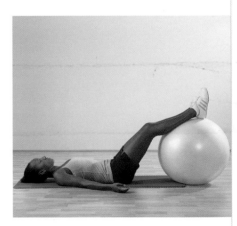

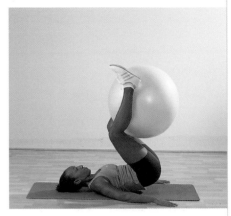

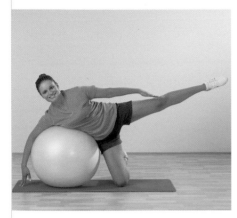

Side leg-lift (see pages 46–47)

Wall squat (see pages 58–59)

Splits stretch (see pages 84–85)

Lower ab curl (see pages 44–45)

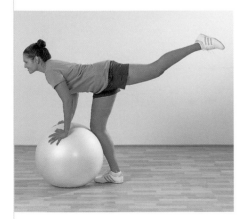

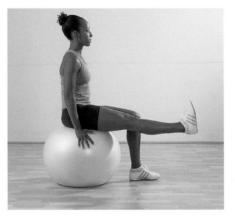

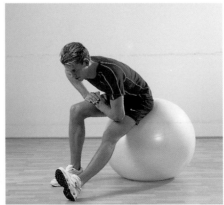

Butt kick (see pages 50–51)

Quad toner (see pages 56–57)

Hamstring hang (see pages 78–79)

Cool-down: leg elevation (see page 19)

The 45-minute Routine

You can give yourself a thorough workout in 45 minutes, so if you can't always fit in all the exercises, do this routine at least two or three times a week. Follow the recommendations for repetitions and sets given with each exercise. If you want to save time, do fewer repetitions or sets, but make sure you tone and stretch each side of your body evenly. Don't worry if you can't do it in 45 minutes at first—you will speed up as you get used to the moves.

This routine is designed to help you tone and stretch a range of muscles in the body, but try to complete the full workout from time to time so that you are familiar with all the exercises.

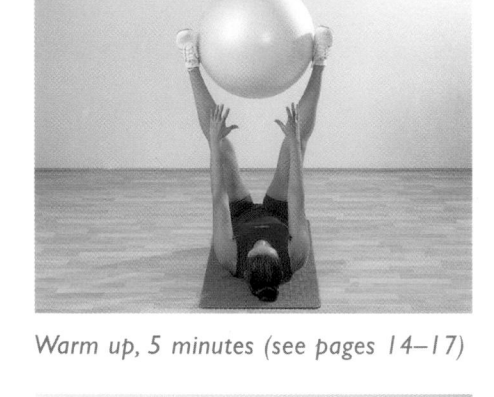
Warm up, 5 minutes (see pages 14–17)

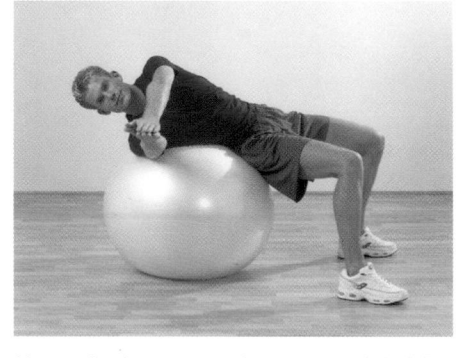
Upper-body rotation (see pages 24–25)

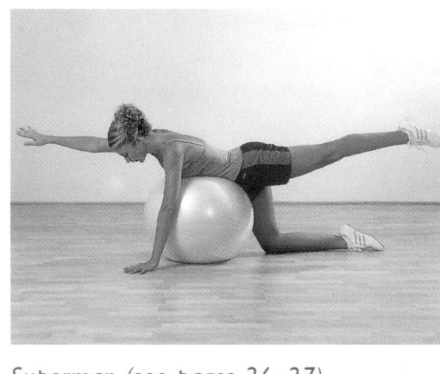
Superman (see pages 26–27)

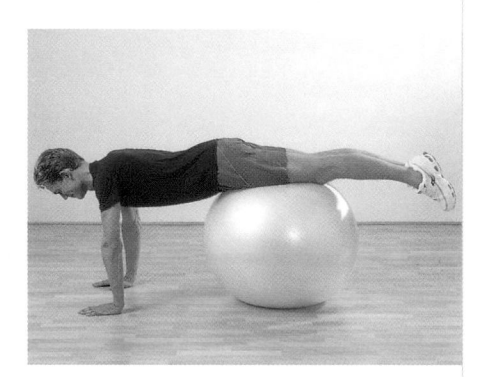
Push-up perfecter (see pages 28–29)

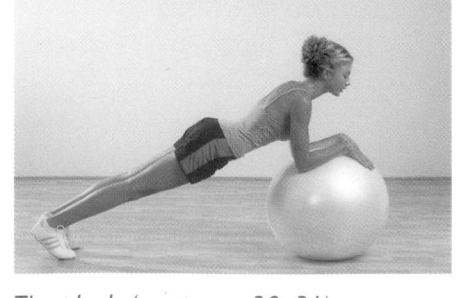
The plank (see pages 30–31)

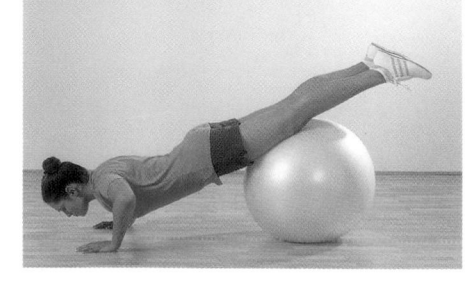
Push-up (see pages 34–35)

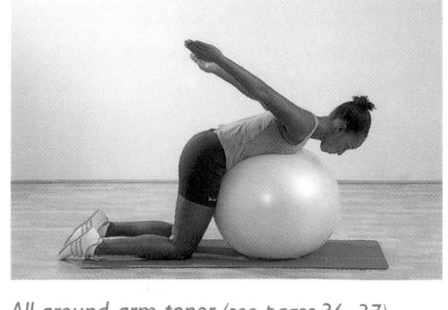
All-around arm toner (see pages 36–37)

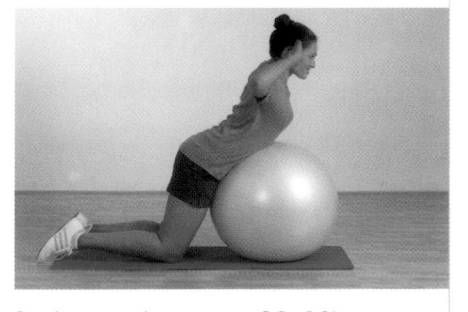
Back toner (see pages 38–39)

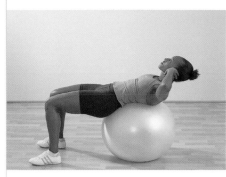

Basic ab curl (see pages 40–41)

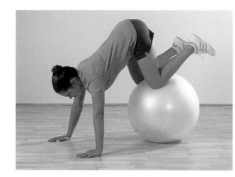

Ab contraction (see pages 42–43)

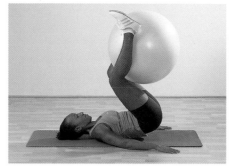

Lower ab curl (see pages 44–45)

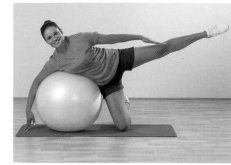

Side leg-lift (see pages 46–47)

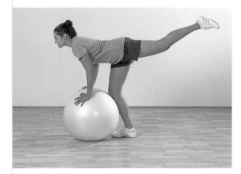

Butt kick (see pages 50–51)

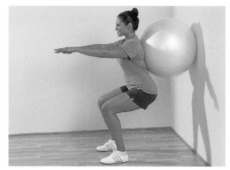

Wall squat (see pages 58–59)

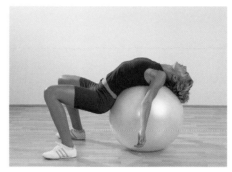

Back archery (see pages 68–69)

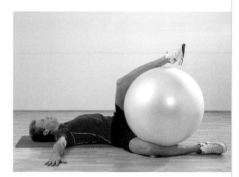

Lower-back twister (see pages 74–75)

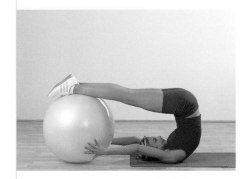

Yoga bridge (see pages 76–77)

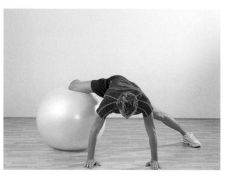

Inner-thigh thinner (see pages 82–83)

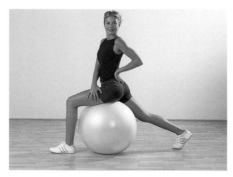

Splits stretch (see pages 84–85)

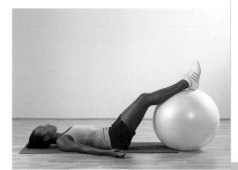

Cool-down: leg elevation (see page 19)

THE 45-MINUTE ROUTINE

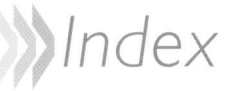

Index

AUTHOR'S ACKNOWLEDGMENTS
Thank you to all at Carroll & Brown for their professionalism and attention to detail.

CARROLL & BROWN WOULD LIKE TO THANK:
Models
Bronwyn Belcher, Peter Hvass, Karen Lanson, Dionne Wright

Hair and make-up
Jeseama Owen

Female models' clothes supplied by:

sweaty**Betty**
833 Fulham Road
London
SW6 5HQ
+44 (0)800 1693889
www.sweatyBetty.com